Through the Seasons

A Johns Hopkins Press Health Book

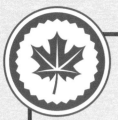

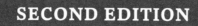
SECOND EDITION

THROUGH
THE
SEASONS

ACTIVITIES FOR
Memory-Challenged Adults
and Their Caregivers

Cynthia R. Green, PhD
Joan Beloff, ACC, ALA, CDP

Foreword by Peter V. Rabins, MD, MPH

JOHNS HOPKINS UNIVERSITY PRESS

Baltimore

Johns Hopkins University Press
2715 North Charles Street
Baltimore, Maryland 21218-4363
www.press.jhu.edu

Library of Congress Cataloging-in-Publication Data

Names: Green, Cynthia R., author. | Beloff, Joan, 1953– author.
Title: Through the seasons : activities for memory-challenged adults and
    their caregivers / Cynthia R. Green, PhD, Joan Beloff, ACC, ALA, CDP ;
    foreword by Peter V. Rabins, MD, MPH.
Description: Second edition. | Baltimore : John Hopkins University Press,
    2020. | Series: A Johns Hopkins Press health book.
Identifiers: LCCN 2019016215 | ISBN 9781421436463 (hardcover) |
    ISBN 1421436469 (hardcover) | ISBN 9781421436470 (paperback) |
    ISBN 1421436477 (paperback) | ISBN 9781421436487 (electronic) |
    ISBN 1421436485 (electronic)
Subjects: LCSH: Memory disorders—Patients—Rehabilitation. |
    Dementia—Patients—Rehabilitation. | Memory disorders in old
    age—Patients—Rehabilitation. | Caregivers.
Classification: LCC RC394.M46 G74 2020 | DDC 616.8/3—dc23
LC record available at https://lccn.loc.gov/2019016215

A catalog record for this book is available from the British Library.

All photographs are © iStockphoto except on the following pages:
23, © Susanna Cesareo / Shutterstock.com; 29, © Alina Reynbakh /
Shutterstock.com; 33, © www.YourFleece.com.

"Casey at the Bat" on pages 94–95 is from www.poets.org.

*Special discounts are available for bulk purchases of this book. For more information,
please contact Special Sales at 410-516-6936 or specialsales@press.jhu.edu.*

Johns Hopkins University Press uses environmentally friendly book materials,
including recycled text paper that is composed of at least 30 percent post-consumer
waste, whenever possible.

To those living with memory challenge and those caring for them. We hope the experiences offered in this book, and those that you find for yourself along the way as you use them, will create moments together that bring joy, meaning, and connection.

CONTENTS

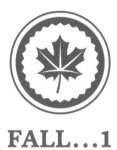

FOREWORD

Peter V. Rabins, MD, MPH

When I first became interested in the care of people with dementia forty years ago, I read an article by geriatric psychiatrist Dr. Jack Weinberg entitled, "What Do I Say to My Mother When I Have Nothing to Say?" In it, Dr. Weinberg describes the frustration he experienced when talking with his mother, who was cognitively impaired and living in a long-term facility. To him, these conversations were contrived and repetitive, and he quickly ran out of new things to say. His feelings of frustration and helplessness totally changed once he realized that the most important aspect of talking with his mother was the pleasure she experienced when engaged in a conversation, not the specific content of their conversation.

Dr. Weinberg's realization made his daily talks with his mother much more meaningful for both of them. This insight helped him enjoy their interactions as he had before her illness, and this, in turn, improved her mood and sense of well-being. Reading his article helped me appreciate the importance of maintaining social engagement for people with dementia.

As Cynthia Green and Joan Beloff demonstrate in *Through the Seasons*, we've learned a lot since Dr. Weinberg's article. Most importantly, perhaps, are the ideas that it *does* matter what we talk about and do when we interact with people who are experiencing dementia and that it *is* important to fit the content of verbal interactions and physical activity to the person's abilities and strengths as well as the specifics of their lives. But underlying the approach of *Through the Seasons* is the insight that Dr. Weinberg experienced: Maintaining meaningful human contact with people experiencing dementia is important no matter how ill they are.

Through the Seasons beautifully balances a discussion of the principles underlying this approach with specific, practical, and reasonable guidance on how to actually do it. With Cynthia Green and Joan Beloff's guidance, staying focused on the primary goal of dementia care—maximizing the quality of life of people with dementia—becomes achievable.

It is easy to underestimate the skill that it takes to reach this goal. What I particularly like about *Through the Seasons* is that the specificity of its suggestions helps get us over the hump of initiating and sustaining meaningful conversations and activities with people experiencing a range of cognitive disabilities. This is an important first step in developing the skills needed by both the professional care provider and the family caregiver. For the professional, the book provides a range of suggestions, advice, and templates—a roadmap, if you will—for refining their skills and helping them personalize interactions with those they are caring for. For the caregiver of a family member with dementia, *Through the Seasons* will help get past the barriers identified by Dr. Weinberg as well as help identify the steps they can take to provide the stimulation that is so important for the person with dementia's quality of life.

This new edition is notable for its greater emphasis on linking the lifelong experiences of people with dementia to the content of their current interactions. This emphasis on care recipients' ethnic and experiential backgrounds as well as their values and wants addresses the worldwide trend of increasing ethnic diversity.

A combination of increasing longevity and increasing emigration means that people with dementia in any single location, and the professionals who are providing their care, are now more diverse than was true in the past. In addition, a worldwide trend towards decreasing family size means that family caregivers will be increasingly unavailable. *Through the Seasons* provides a needed guide to address these trends.

The thread that ties together the strands of guidance and understanding contained in *Through the Seasons* is the word "joy"—joy in those who are experiencing dementia, joy in those who are providing care to them, and the joy and satisfaction that comes from knowing that there are tools available to help those who want to improve the care of people with dementia. By providing a practical guide to helping people achieve the satisfaction that comes from having enjoyable interactions and accomplishing pleasurable tasks, *Through the Seasons* has played and will continue to play an important role in maximizing quality of life of people with dementia.

PREFACE

It is difficult to believe that more than a decade has passed since the publication of the first edition of *Through the Seasons*.

The idea for the book initially arose from our frustration at the time with the quality and tone of the available cognitive-stimulation resources for individuals with memory loss and their caregivers. While the evidence suggested that such programs could be beneficial, much of the material we found was limited and, in many instances, childish and demeaning in approach. It was our intention to provide activities that offered fulfilling engagement while fostering opportunities for continued meaningful connection and communication between those with memory disorders and the families and professionals who cared for them. It has been both gratifying and humbling to hear from the many families and colleagues who have found this collection of activities helpful and inspiring.

Over the past decade, much has changed in the field of dementia care. Among other things, we have seen scientific advances in dementia management, increased acceptance of person-centered approaches to care, and a growing availability of cognitive-stimulation programs for both institutional and home care settings. We are pleased to have the chance to update the original edition of this book to include new information and materials that reflect this progress.

In this second edition, you will find:

- An updated introduction, covering the rationale behind the program in addition to new information about using the activities in a home or institutional setting.

- Additional activities in each section, along with expanded "Let's Talk About…" and "Let's Try…" prompts for each activity.

- An integrated multicultural approach that offers more activities across different traditions and diverse backgrounds.

- An updated resource section.

It is an honor to have this latest edition available as a companion to Nancy Mace and Peter Rabins's seminal work, *The 36-Hour Day*. Their classic guide remains a favorite that we have long admired and always recommend.

We hope this latest edition of *Through the Seasons* brings many moments of joy, meaning, and connection to the lives of all those it touches. It is our sincerest wish that this book will continue to make it easier to share history and create new moments together. We look forward to hearing about the many ways you use the program and make the experiences your own.

Here's to many wonderful memories, both old and new.

INTRODUCTION

Living with dementia can at times be a challenge, for both those facing memory loss and those who care for them. As professionals, we have witnessed the struggle of our clients and their families to stay connected, engaged, and active in the face of the changes that result from memory disorders and their progression.

Dementia and related disorders impact the lives of those affected and those who care for them in countless, ever-changing ways. Even early on, short-term memory changes can make it difficult to remain independent at work and across activities such as volunteering, traveling, managing finances, and recreational pursuits. Someone who loved to cook, for example, may no longer be able to follow the steps of a recipe or work the stove safely on their own. It can be challenging to find activities that fill the time in ways that feel meaningful to all involved. In addition, the disease often takes a toll on communication, with a person having more difficulty finding words or framing thoughts. A person with dementia may find it increasingly harder to participate in conversations at the dinner table, talk on the phone, or take part in social events. These communication challenges can lead to frustration, withdrawal, and isolation from family, friends, and the community. In turn, these changes in opportunity and connection can diminish the self-esteem and sense of worth of the person with dementia.

Yet current research shows that continued engagement—physical, mental, and social— can make a significant, positive difference in the experience of those living with dementia. *Through the Seasons* offers a program that helps persons living with memory loss and those who care for them do just that. The platform uses enriching activities, discussion topics, and photographs, each tied to a different season of the year, to foster conversation and shared experiences. With prompts that allow you to adapt the activities to different ability levels, *Through the Seasons* is an indispensable solution to the question of "what to do" together to maintain well-being and connection.

CURRENT RESEARCH IN DEMENTIA CARE

First developed over a decade ago, the *Through the Seasons* program continues to use a multi-sensory approach to engaging persons with dementia in cognitively stimulating activities that promote well-being, self-worth, and connection. This latest edition has been updated to reflect scientific and cultural advances since the program was first released, including the following modifications.

Wellness Approach

Research shows that engaging in activities that promote well-being, such as getting regular exercise, eating well, and managing stress, contribute to a better quality of life for those living with dementia. Some interventions, such as regular aerobic exercise and mindfulness meditation, have additionally been linked in studies to slowing disease progression. *Through the Seasons* integrates wellness across the different activities suggested in the program.

Person-Centered Focus

Perhaps the greatest shift in the memory care culture since the initial release of *Through the Seasons* is the widespread acceptance of a person-centered focus in care planning and provision. Defined as "a philosophy of care built around the needs of the individual and contingent upon knowing the person through an interpersonal relationship" (Fazio, Pace, Flinner, et al. 2018), a person-centered focus is the lynchpin of the recently released *Alzheimer's Association Dementia Care Practice Recommendations*. The *Through the Seasons* program has taken a person-centered approach since its inception, highlighting the person's unique interests, background, likes, and dislikes to inform the way in which the activities are chosen and done together. As stated in the original introduction, the activities suggested "provide an opportunity for self-expression and increased sense of self-worth." This latest version continues to promote a person-centered approach—in the guide for using the program, in the wide range of choices on how to tailor each experience for the individual, and in the inclusion of many multicultural prompts and activities.

Cognitive Stimulation

Cognitive stimulation therapy, especially in the company of other therapies, has been found to improve thinking and quality of life for persons with memory loss. In one of the most exhaustive reviews of the science to date, the *Lancet* Commission on Dementia Prevention, Intervention, and Care concluded that cognitive stimulation therapy is "the psychological approach with the strongest evidence for improving cognition" (Livingston, Sommerlad, Orgeta, et al. 2017). *Through the Seasons* is, at its heart, a program that provides persons living with dementia the opportunities for continued cognitive and social stimulation. These in turn support ongoing communication and meaningful connections to family, friends, and community, as well as self-worth and personhood. Designed primarily for use at home by the affected individual and their care partners, this program adapts easily and is frequently used in group programs in residential and community settings.

REFERENCES

Fazio S., Pace D., Flinner J., Kallmyer B. *The Fundamentals of Person-Centered Care for Individuals with Dementia*. Gerontologist. 2018 Jan 18;58(suppl 1):S10–S19. doi: 10.1093/geront/gnx122. PubMed PMID: 29361064.

Fazio S., Pace D., Maslow K., et al. *Alzheimer's Association Dementia Care Practice Recommendations*. Gerontologist. 2018 Jan 18;58(suppl 1):S1–S9. doi: 10.1093/geront/gnx182. PubMed PMID: 29361074.

Livingston G., Sommerlad A., Orgeta V., et al. *Dementia Prevention, Intervention, and Care*. Lancet. 2017 Dec 16;390(10113): 2673-2734. doi: 10.1016/S0140-6736 (17)31363-6. Epub 2017 Jul 20. Review. PubMed PMID: 28735855.

THROUGH THE SEASONS: ABOUT THE PROGRAM

In *Through the Seasons*, you will find a series of simple, common experiences to explore together. These experiences are grouped into four sections or themes, each focusing on a season of the year: fall, winter, spring, and summer. The book uses an enriched, multisensory approach, highlighting a collaborative exploration that engages the five senses and allowing for adaptation across levels of interest and ability to achieve successful engagement.

You will find a total of 32 experiences to choose from, with 8 in each theme. Each experience in *Through the Seasons* offers:

- **A photograph** chosen for its simplicity and illustration of the experience in order to stimulate discussion and memories. For example, in the summer section, you will find the experience of eating ice cream, a common and popular summer activity.

- **An introductory prompt** to begin conversation about the experience, such as "Ice cream tastes good on a hot summer day."

- **"Let's Talk About…"** questions to guide further discussion and exploration. As part of the summer experience featuring ice cream, you might talk about favorite ice-cream flavors or toppings.

- **"Let's Try…"** ideas that offer a wide range of suggested multisensory activities to enrich and more fully engage together in the experience. For example, you may decide to explore the "ice cream" experience together by having an old-fashioned ice-cream social with a group of family or friends or take a trip to a local ice-cream store.

- **"Let's Make…"** activities for each theme, with additional instructions, such as recipes, directions for craft projects, and more, to aid in bringing the activity to your setting.

Each experience is laid out across two pages so that two people can easily look at them together. Try sitting side by side as you look at the book. Use nonverbal cues, such as gentle touch or pointing to details in the photos, to help guide discussion and give direction. As for all of us, gentle physical closeness can be reassuring for persons with dementia, especially when staying focused is a challenge.

GETTING STARTED WITH THE PROGRAM

Choose Your Path

Before using the *Through the Seasons* program, take the time to look over all of the experiences that are offered. Decide how you want to use the program materials. The program can be used in endless ways, offering tremendous flexibility in what you do with it over time.

For example, you may first wish to read the whole book together, using only the "Let's Talk About…" prompts to foster conversation. Or you may prefer to begin slowly, starting with the experiences that reflect the current season of the year. You may even choose to focus on only one activity at a time, depending on individual needs or the setting in which you are using the program. When using the "Let's Try…" or "Let's Make…" activities, think together about what you both may enjoy so that you can plan accordingly to gather the needed materials or arrange for trips in advance.

Personalize the Experience

Once you have decided how you will begin to use the *Through the Seasons* program, think about how you might adapt the suggested activities to further personalize the experience for any specific needs, interests, likes, and dislikes. For example, someone who always enjoyed gardening may enjoy experiences that highlight nature, such as walks outdoors or looking through gardening magazines. You may find that other ideas come to mind that will allow you to deepen the experiences or lead you toward other paths to explore together. These are all welcome ways of using the *Through the Seasons* materials.

Establish the Setting

Next, think ahead about the setting in which you will enjoy the *Through the Seasons* program together. Work together in a location which is quiet, where you are unlikely to be interrupted or distracted. Persons with memory loss may have a harder time maintaining focus, and a quieter setting will increase your chances of engaging together in a meaningful and enjoyable way.

Establish the Time

Choose a time to enjoy the program together when you will be able to fully engage without feeling rushed or constrained. Allow yourself the flexibility to adjust according to the mood and pace of the day so that the time you spend together doing the activities is enjoyable. For example, if late morning tends to be a time when the person living with dementia is calmer and more alert, establish the routine of using the program around that time. You can use the program as part of your daily care plan as a way of including meaningful activities each day (see the Sample Daily Care Plan on page xix for more guidance).

Organize Your Materials
Be sure that you have gathered all the materials you will need before embarking on the experiences you have chosen to do together. You can organize them ahead of time in a special area or in a small box set aside for that purpose. Having the necessary items laid out beforehand will make it easier for you to stay focused on enjoying the activity together, rather than interrupting the experience by having to go get items. Work together as much as possible in organizing the materials for your activity, including the person with dementia in tasks that can help them be part of the process.

BEST PRACTICES AND TIPS FOR USING *THROUGH THE SEASONS*

The creative activities suggested in this book provide a great opportunity for individuals to express themselves and build self-worth. How can everyone get the most out of the *Through the Seasons* program? Here are some best practices and tips to optimize your experience using these materials together.

Choose Activities That Foster Self-Expression and Confidence
Matching the individual's current level of ability to the activities will allow them to gain the most benefit. Persons facing memory loss will vary in their ability to participate in the suggested activities. This may be due to individual

differences, such as sensory changes or mood state, as well as the impact of the memory disorder itself. In addition, the kinds of activities that engage someone will change as their condition progresses. Be sure to select activities appropriate to where the person is "at" when you are doing the program together. Prepare to modify activities to best meet the individual's current level of ability, whether over the course of a few days or a few years. Doing so will ensure that everyone gets the most out of the program.

Allow Independence
Let the person with memory loss be as independent as possible during the activity. Focus on being partners in the experience rather than leading them through it. Think about doing the activity "with" and not "for" them. Keep any interference with the activity or experience to a minimum, reserved for times when it appears that the experience will lead to harm or upset. Do not be concerned with the outcome—that is not, after all, the true goal. Rather, focus on the quality of the time you are having together—the opportunity to share things from the past and to create something new. Interrupting the process to straighten a photograph or correct how something is glued isn't necessary and may diminish the memory-challenged person's sense of accomplishment and desire to participate.

Set Appropriate Expectations
As you do the activities together, always be respectful and protect the dignity of the individual. For example, invite your loved one to join you in an activity, rather than telling them to do it. Keep in mind that just because someone is living with memory changes doesn't mean they have changed their minds about the things they like and dislike. Choose respectfully, selecting experiences they might have enjoyed previously. While it's fine to try something new together, do not force participation. It is okay to not enjoy an activity,

no matter who we are! If the individual has difficulty expressing themselves, try keeping a journal of what experiences they seem to like or dislike. You can then use what you learn from the recorded information to guide your choice of experiences in the future. Finally, be realistic about what you are trying to accomplish together. If you attempt activities that are too difficult, you will both be frustrated and disappointed. Likewise, activities that are too simple may feel demeaning and discouraging.

Keep It Safe

Whenever you engage someone living with memory loss in an activity, you must perform a safety assessment. Memory disorders can often affect an individual's judgement about his or her own safety and ability. Therefore, you must take responsibility for making sound decisions and taking precautions to ensure that the person can safely participate in any planned activity. Before introducing an activity, look for any safety challenges it may raise. For example, can the person safely perform the physical activity required, such as walking across a lawn or cutting up apples? What steps do you need to take to ensure that they are protected from accidents while cooking, or using scissors? If you are preparing for a group activity such as an ice-cream social, what dietary restrictions do you need to consider?

Once you have reviewed all the possible safety issues associated with an experience, think through what you need to do to modify the activity to make it safe. For example, you may need to pre-slice the apples if you are making applesauce or provide sugar-free ice cream and toppings if any of the persons attending your ice-cream social follow a sugar-free diet.

Encourage Reminiscing

Many of the experiences included in *Through the Seasons* are designed to foster reminiscing. This can tap memories that are still very much alive for the individual living with dementia. In most memory disorders, long-term memories such as those about childhood or early adulthood are accessible and well-preserved. Sharing such stories gives the individual a chance to reflect and feel good about the many contributions they made over their lifetime. What a wonderful chance for younger family members, new caregivers, and others to learn about their history, traditions, and accomplishments. We hope you will take advantage of these opportunities, for example, using personal articles in the memory boxes or family photos in the collages to stimulate conversation and prompt the individual to share tales and special memories from the past. Write down the memories shared so that you can talk about them again at a later time or share them with family and friends.

Communication: Use the "Three Cs"

Changes in communication ability—to either verbalize or understand what is being said—are frequently seen in memory loss, especially as the disease progresses. Such difficulties in communicating with those around us can be frustrating and depressing and lead to increased isolation. It can be easy to mistake communication challenges for a lack of interest or cooperation, when really, the person with memory loss simply cannot easily follow what you are saying.

A tried-and-true best practice for enhancing communication with those with memory loss is the "Three Cs":

- **Calm.** First, maintain *calm* in your voice. Use a steady, reassuring tone. Doing so will set a welcoming, encouraging environment for the activities. Keep in mind that the feelings expressed in your voice are as important as the words you say. Try to maintain this sense of calm even when things may not be going exactly as you would like.

- **Concise.** Next, be *concise* with your speech. Use simple words that are concrete and easy to understand. Keep your sentences short and direct so that they will be easy to grasp and follow.

- **Consistent.** Finally, be *consistent* with your choice of words and directions. Using the same phrasing throughout your communications can make it easier for the person facing memory loss to understand your intent and engage in the conversation.

For example, when using the "Let's Talk About…" questions, speak clearly and distinctly in a level and composed manner and keep your wording straightforward. Try to avoid pronouns. Instead of saying, "Here it is," point to the image or object and say, "Here is the ice-cream cone in the picture." Ask only one question at a time, making sure to give the person plenty of time to respond. Do not rush the person, as doing so will only add to the confusion and lead to frustration for everyone. If they do not seem to understand, repeat the question using the same wording. If after a few minutes this still does not work, try rephrasing the question slightly. Above all, remember that it is important for you to be an attentive, good listener and not interrupt the person's thought process.

Over time, you may find that there are changes in the way the person living with memory loss is able to understand and use language. It is not uncommon for someone to use familiar words over and over again, to invent new words to describe common objects, or to have difficulty putting words in the correct sequence. The memory-challenged person may revert to the first language they learned or, at times, seem to be speaking nonsense. Again, if you use the "Three Cs"—remain calm, concise, and consistent in your approach and conversation—it will give both of you a better chance to benefit from the program.

Finally, if you pose a question and do not understand the response, try to tap into the meaning or the emotion behind what is being said. Repeating what was said can often lead to clarification. After repeating, ask the person some follow-up questions to help them further express their thoughts and feelings. The individual's tone of voice or actions might help you understand what they are saying. Try using questions that begin with the words "who," "what," "when," "where," and "how."

Dealing with Frustration
There may be times while using this program when the person living with memory loss seems frustrated, withdrawn, or even agitated. When this happens, first try to understand what may be happening to cause the reaction. Think about what happened before the person became upset and try to identify what might have triggered their response. Perhaps there is something they need that they are having difficulty expressing, such as wanting a drink or needing to go to the bathroom. Or perhaps they are simply—as we all can be at times—not in the mood! Address the problem and then see if you can go on with the activity or discussion. If, however, they continue to seem frustrated or upset, stop and try again at a later time. Above all, stay calm, positive, and reassuring. Try soothing music or touch to help reestablish a calm mood before you move on to something else. Keeping your interactions with the *Through the Seasons* experiences positive and enjoyable will benefit everyone.

USING *THROUGH THE SEASONS* AT HOME

Through the Seasons is designed to enhance your daily routine with meaningful conversations and a variety of activities that you can enjoy together at different times of the year. While no day is ever the same, especially when living with memory loss, it can be helpful to stick to a daily routine that provides structure to the day. The predictability of a routine can be helpful for all of us, especially for those managing memory challenges. Most of us like to know what we will be doing during certain times of the day, as it helps us be prepared and reduces stress. In addition, having a daily plan can make the job of a caregiver easier as well. Finally, if there are several persons involved in caregiving, a care plan can simplify the way you share information and help you maintain routine and structure.

If you aren't sure what daily routine will work best, try starting with what the person's usual habits have typically been. What time would they usually wake up or go to bed? Eat meals? Exercise? What time of day are they most alert, and when are they more fatigued or easily irritated? Account for regularly enjoyed activities as well, such as meeting with friends for a weekly lunch, reading the paper on Sunday mornings, watching a favorite TV show, or attending religious services. Finally, keep in mind their likes, dislikes, strengths, abilities, and interests. From here, you can begin to develop a daily care plan that will help provide focus and structure to the day.

While everyone will have their own routine, we've included a sample daily care plan you can use as a guide. Just remember to stay open and flexible to allow for changes as needed.

Decide when it may be a good opportunity to try different activities, like those found in *Through the Seasons*, at a regular time in the schedule. Choose a time that works best for both of you, when you can focus on enjoying the experience together. If needed, break the experience into smaller steps that can be done one at a time. For example, if working on a collage, you may start by identifying the images you want to use, then cutting them out together the next time, and finally creating the collage together on a third occasion. When you are planning outings, schedule them for the time of day when the person is at their best, and aim to return home before they get too tired.

SAMPLE DAILY CARE PLAN

MORNING
- Wash up, brush teeth, get dressed
- Prepare and eat breakfast
- Do clean-up chores
- Orient to the date, current events
- Morning activity
- Social time with coffee or tea
- Walk or morning exercise

AFTERNOON
- Prepare and eat lunch
- Rest and relax
- Afternoon activity

EVENING
- Prepare and eat dinner
- Evening activity
- Quiet time
- Prepare for bed

USING *THROUGH THE SEASONS* IN A GROUP SETTING

The program provided in *Through the Seasons* can easily be adapted for use in a small group, such as a memory care or day program setting. In fact, working together with others may actually boost the benefit by increasing the memory-challenged individual's level of engagement with the experiences.

In addition to the suggestions above, here are some best practices and tips for using *Through the Seasons* when working with a group.

Think Small and Inclusive
Be thoughtful when selecting participants for a group. First, think "small." Participants will benefit most from this program when the group's size is kept to about 4–6 persons. This allows everyone to work together, but at a pace and rhythm that is inclusive and considerate of individual challenges. Next, invite persons

at similar levels of cognitive ability. This will make it easier to run the activities as a group leader so that, for example, you can better plan outings or manage potential safety issues like using scissors. If possible, select group members who you think might work well together, have similar interests, and enjoy each other's company. Planning to run multiple small groups will allow you to best accommodate everyone's needs so that they can optimally benefit from the program.

Choose Experiences Best Suited to Your Group

When adapting the *Through the Seasons* experiences for group delivery, be sure to opt for discussions and activities that can be best used by your group. We suggest looking over the entire program first, marking those experiences that seem most fitting, both in terms of ability as well as interest. Look for things that can be done together. For example, many of the cooking or craft suggestions would work quite well, while some of the activities that focus on personal history, such as using family photos, may not.

Build Relationships

Delivering *Through the Seasons* in a small group offers a wonderful opportunity to foster social connections between participants. Lead the experiences with a gentle eye towards helping group members build relationships with each other. Try to avoid engagement solely between yourself as the group leader and the individual participants. Rather, encourage group members to connect with each other as they are able to, both verbally and nonverbally. Sharing memories and working together, and even singing old songs or creating art with each other, will provide many opportunities for participants to feel supported and connected to each other in a group setting.

Establish Expectations for Inclusion, Respect, and Dignity

Finally, be sure to set guidelines that are welcoming and inclusive of everyone in the group. Use a calm, consistent manner that makes all group members feel comfortable. Encourage participants to be part of the discussions in the many different ways that they are able to, including movement or other nonverbal means of communicating. Find an avenue for everyone to be part of an activity so that they are all engaged. Allow everyone to work at their own pace and make it clear that your group is a "failure-free" zone, where the goal is being together and enjoying the activity rather than a polished product. Leading with inclusion, respect, and dignity for all will set that expectation for your group and foster an environment where everyone can optimally benefit from the program.

We hope that *Through the Seasons* will bring many wonderful, shared experiences to the lives of memory-challenged individuals and those who care for them. It is our sincerest wish that *Through the Seasons* will make a difference, not only in stimulating old memories but also in creating new ones. We look forward to hearing the many ways in which you use this book and make the experiences and activities your own. Thank you for letting us be part of the process.

Through the Seasons

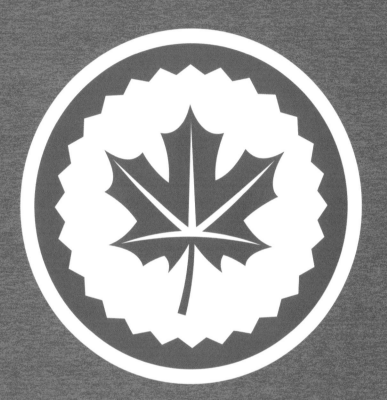

FALL

LET'S TALK ABOUT ...

- Did you ever carve a pumpkin?

- What kinds of faces did you make on the pumpkin?

- Let's name some different ways we eat pumpkin. (If needed, prompt the person by beginning to name some ways we eat pumpkin, such as pumpkin pie, bread, soup, etc.)

- What is your favorite dish to make with pumpkin?

- Did you ever eat pumpkin soup or pumpkin pie?

- What other kinds of squash do you like to eat? For example, acorn, butternut, zucchini?

- Did you ever go to a pumpkin patch? Can you tell me about it?

LET'S TRY ...

- Making pumpkin treats, such as pumpkin bread or muffins, using a packaged mix or cookbook recipe. You can also make or buy pumpkin-shaped cookies to decorate as jack-o'-lanterns with orange and black icing.

- Roasting and eating pumpkin seeds.

- Carving a pumpkin together and placing a battery-operated candle inside.

- Reading poems about pumpkins or the fall together. Try moving while reading the poems, or try talking about what memories the poems bring up. You can find poems ("Theme in Yellow" by Carl Sandburg is a favorite!) on websites such as www.poets.org or www.poetry foundation.org.

- Making a pumpkin beanbag toss. Get 2–3 plastic jack-o'-lanterns and several small beanbags. Place them on the floor a few feet away from your chairs. Toss the beanbags into the pumpkins.

- Decorating a pumpkin using drip art. Purchase different water-based paints, and use brushes to "drip" the paint on the pumpkin. You can also decorate the pumpkin using yarn, buttons, wiggly eyes, and markers.

- Eating spaghetti squash. Purchase spiral-cut spaghetti squash and sauté with olive oil or butter. Add vegetables, sauces, and parmesan cheese, as desired.

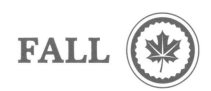

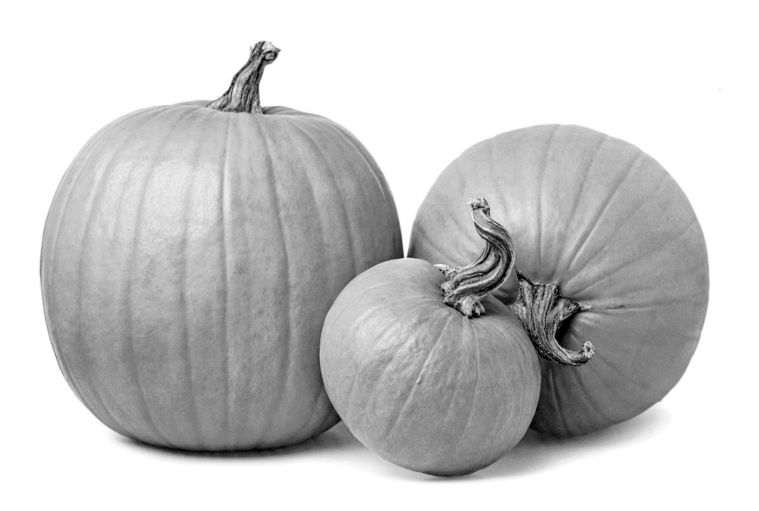

Pumpkins are a sign of fall.

LET'S MAKE CURRIED SQUASH SOUP

Make a pureed squash soup to enjoy together. If desired, omit the curry spice for a milder flavored soup.

You Will Need:

- 4 small yellow potatoes, peeled and cubed
- 2 pounds butternut squash, peeled and cubed
- 2 medium apples, peeled and cubed
- 1 medium yellow onion, chopped
- 1 quart chicken or vegetable broth

- ½ teaspoon powdered ginger
- ½ teaspoon cumin
- ¼ teaspoon ground nutmeg
- 1 teaspoon curry powder (*optional*)
- 1 teaspoon butter
- Salt and pepper to taste

Instructions

- In a large pot, cover the squash with water and boil until tender. Drain and reserve the liquid.
- In the same pot, add the butter. When the butter has melted, add the onions and sauté until caramelized.
- Return the squash to the pot. Add potatoes, apples, broth, and spices.

- Add the water you used to boil the squash to the pot, adding more water as needed to fill the pot to the top. Bring to a boil.
- Simmer at a low temperature for one hour.
- Remove from heat and let cool.
- Puree soup to the desired consistency using an immersion blender.

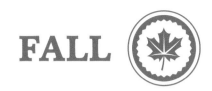
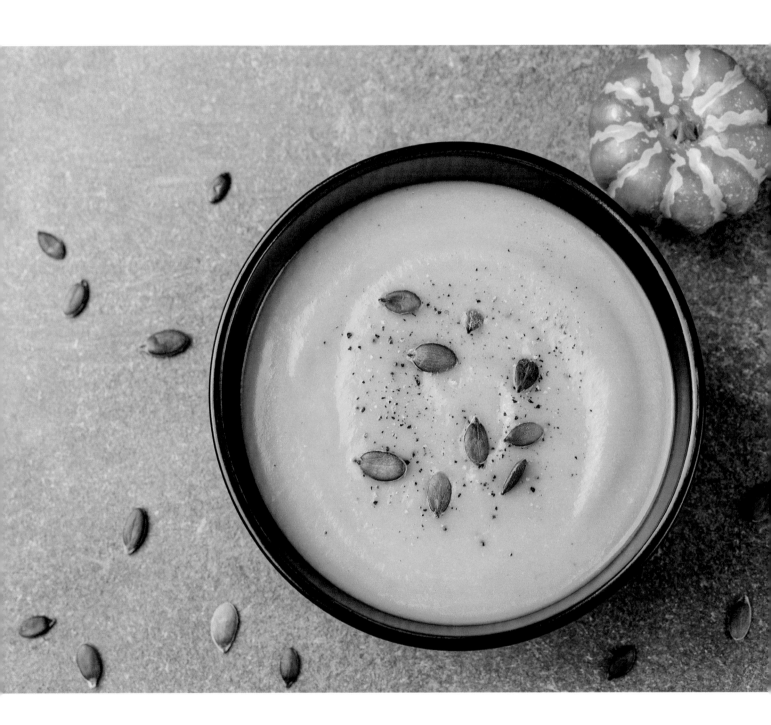

LET'S TALK ABOUT . . .

▶ Did you ever go apple picking? Where would you go to pick apples?

▶ Did you ever smell apples baking? Let's talk about what that smells like.

▶ Did you ever make applesauce? How did you do it?

▶ What do apples make you think about?

▶ Did you have an apple tree in your yard? In your neighborhood?

▶ What different apple tastes and textures do you like? (Sweet, tart, crunchy, soft, etc.)

▶ Many traditions have special recipes that use apples. What family recipes do you have that use apples?

▶ What are your favorite ways to eat apples? (Sliced, with honey, baked, as a sauce, with peanut butter, etc.)

LET'S TRY . . .

▶ Naming different kinds of apples together. (Gala, Macoun, Red Delicious, Granny Smith, Empire, McIntosh, Honeycrisp, etc.)

▶ Making or eating baked apples, apple crisp, or apple pie.

▶ Making applesauce. You can either make the applesauce from scratch using a recipe from a cookbook, or you can warm ready-made applesauce on the stovetop, adding spices such as ground cinnamon and clove.

▶ Visiting a local farm to walk through the orchards and pick apples together.

▶ Going to the grocery store or a farmer's market to look at the different kinds of apples.

▶ Cutting up and eating apples, dipping them in honey or chocolate. Listen to the sounds you make as you eat them together.

▶ Drinking apple cider. Try warming the cider with mulling spices on the stovetop.

▶ Singing songs about apples, such as "Johnny Appleseed," "Don't Sit Under the Apple Tree," and "Little Green Apples."

▶ Writing a short poem together about apples and the fall.

▶ Making apple prints. Cut apples into varying shapes. Place different color water-based paints in several shallow dishes. Dip the apples in the paint and use them to "print" on paper, using the different apple shapes and paints to create an art piece together.

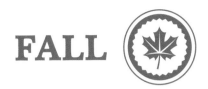

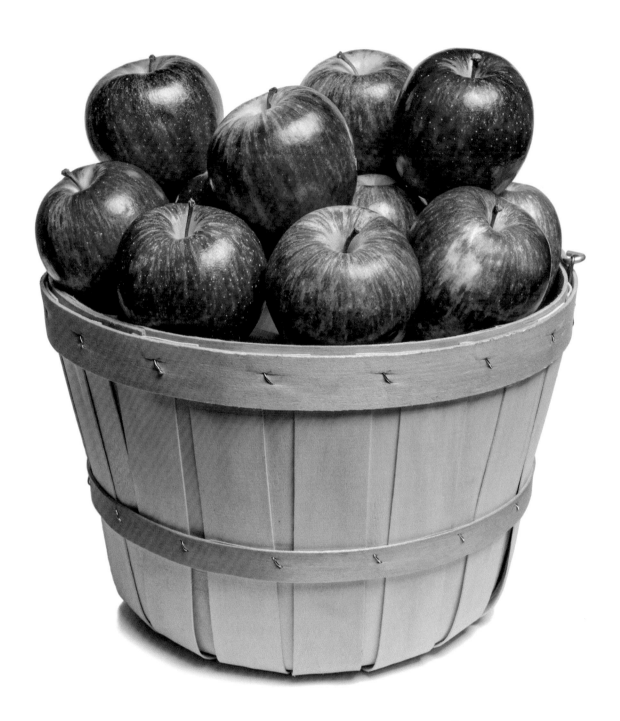

Apples are crisp and crunchy.

LET'S TALK ABOUT ...

- What was your favorite Halloween costume as a child? What can you tell me about it?

- What are some scary stories or ghost stories you remember?

- What traditions for celebrating ghosts or ancestors did your family have? What are some special foods you would make or eat? Who would you celebrate with?

- Did you ever make a haunted house?

- Did you ever bob for apples? Or carve a pumpkin to make a jack-o'-lantern?

- What other holidays would you dress in costumes for as a child?

- What is your favorite candy?

LET'S TRY ...

- Naming different kinds of candies and treats given out for Halloween.

- Reading or listening to ghost stories together.

- Making or purchasing offerings for the Day of the Dead, a traditional Mexican holiday. You can purchase or make traditional baked goods (sugar skulls, *pan de muertos*) or other favorite treats. You can also decorate an altar to honor the dead, using marigolds, electric candles, photos, and other items.

- Having a Hungry Ghost Festival, a traditional Buddhist and Taoist holiday celebrated in the 7th month of the Chinese calendar across Asia. You can make "ghosts," decorate a room with Chinese lanterns and other decorations, listen to traditional Chinese music, eat Asian foods and treats, and make "Hungry Ghost money" (*see activity*) as an offering.

- Watching classic films or TV shows about witches, such as *Bell, Book and Candle*; *Bewitched*; *The Witches of Eastwick*; or *The Wizard of Oz*.

- Singing along to Halloween songs (you can find collections of songs online).

- Having a Halloween party for family and friends. Decorate the room with Halloween-themed decor and have Halloween-themed activities, such as creating masks or witch hats with Halloween stamps or stickers, apple printmaking, or painting small pumpkins or squash. Serve different Halloween treats, such as mulled cider, candies safe for your loved ones (you can slice them into smaller servings if needed), and pumpkin- or ghost-shaped treats.

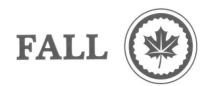

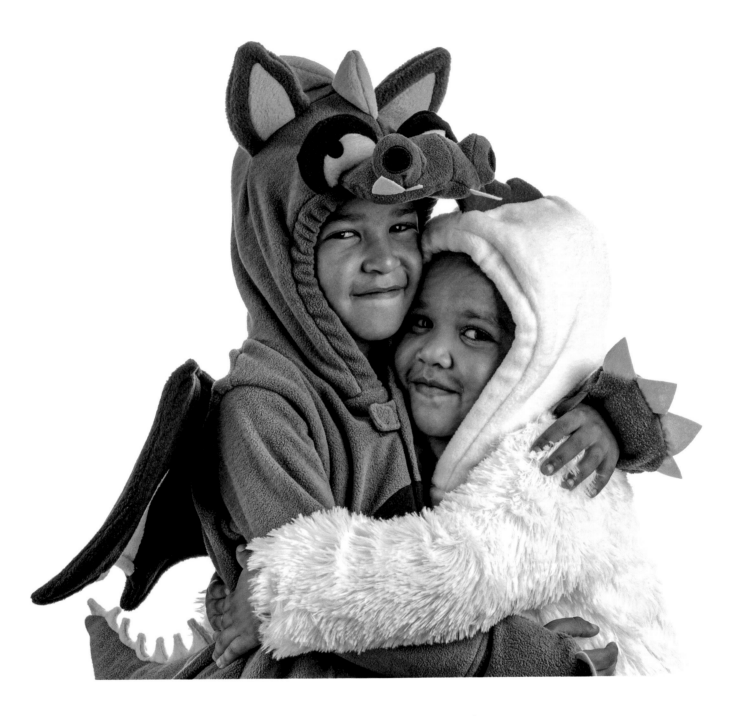

I like to see the children dressed up in costumes.

LET'S MAKE "HUNGRY GHOST MONEY"

The Hungry Ghost Festival is a traditional Buddhist and Taoist holiday celebrated across China and other Asian countries. Held on the 15th day of the 7th month on the Chinese calendar, the celebrations often take place across the entire month, known as the Ghost Month.

The Hungry Ghost Festival marks a time of year when the deceased are thought to be restless and visiting the living. Offerings of food, joss paper "money" and "gold," as well as musical and theatrical performances, are provided to pay respect to, comfort, and guide the spirits back to their rightful place.

Making "Hungry Ghost money" can be a fun and simple creative project you can do together, whether or not it is your tradition to celebrate the Hungry Ghost Festival.

You can find more information and other activity ideas for the Hungry Ghost Festival online. A favorite resource is http://www.chineseamericanfamily.com/hungry-ghost-festival.

You Will Need (you can purchase these items at a crafts store or online):

- Paper, either the traditionally used joss paper or construction or craft paper

- Scissors (safety scissors as needed)

- Water-based nontoxic ink pads and Asian, currency, and other theme-appropriate rubber stamps

- Nontoxic markers, assorted colors

- Theme-appropriate stickers (*optional*)

Instructions

- Cut the paper into currency-sized rectangles. You can do this together or you can cut the paper before you begin.

- Create the "Hungry Ghost money" by decorating the paper with the rubber stamps and markers. If desired, simplify this step by using theme-appropriate stickers.

- Talk about the Hungry Ghost Festival and the cultural meaning behind the holiday as you make the "Hungry Ghost money."

- Use your "Hungry Ghost money" at a Hungry Ghost Festival celebration or simply for decoration.

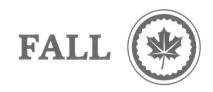

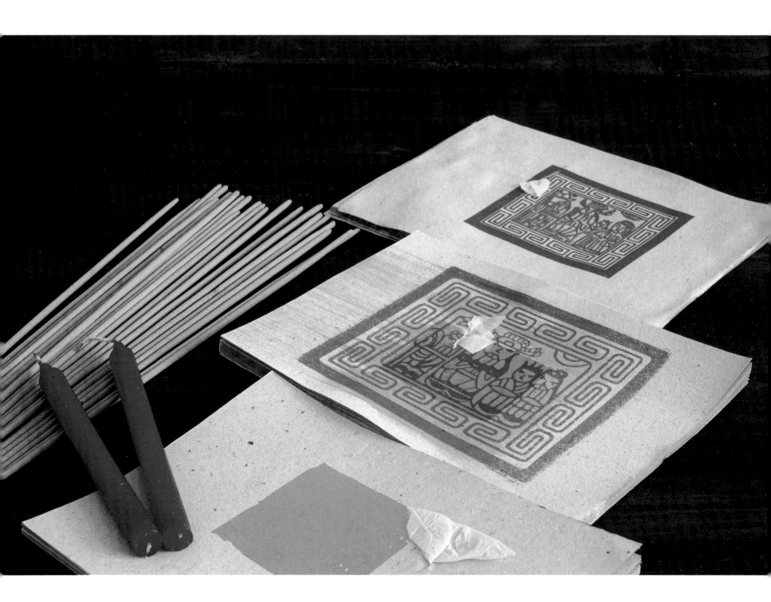

LET'S TALK ABOUT...

- Do you ever sit and watch the leaves fall from the trees?

- Do you like to rake leaves?

- What kinds of games would you play in the fallen leaves?

- What do the smells of fall remind you of?

- Do you remember the smell of leaves burning?

- What are your favorite fall colors?

- What are some colors that leaves change to in the fall?

- Do you like to eat nuts? Do you like to eat them plain, roasted, or salted?

LET'S TRY...

- Naming different colors the leaves turn in fall.

- Naming different kinds of trees. (Oak, chestnut, poplar, beech, pine, fir, cedar, maple, cypress, etc.)

- Taking a drive through a local park or forest to see the fall foliage.

- Collecting leaves and making a collage.

- Raking leaves.

- Naming different tree nuts (almonds, pine nuts, cashews, walnuts, chestnuts, acorns, pistachios, etc.) and talking about how they taste and which are our favorites.

- Taking a walk outside to look at the leaves and talk about what season it is, how the leaves look, and how they may change next.

- Walking through the leaves, kicking through them, or throwing them up in the air.

- Making cookies in the shape of leaves and decorating them with fall-colored icing.

- Looking through photography books together that feature images of fall scenes, forests, and so on.

- Creating a fall sensory box. Place different items that are found during the fall (pine needles, nuts, leaves, small twigs or branches, etc.) in a box. Use the box to experience and recall things about the fall season together.

- Playing a leaf-matching game. Use 3 × 5 index cards, rubber stamps in the shape of leaves, colored markers in fall colors, and/or leaf images from the internet or magazines to create a deck of cards where you have pairs of cards with the same identical leaf images on them. You can play a matching game where you place the cards face down and take turns finding the matching pair of leaf cards by turning two cards face up at a time. Or you can simplify the game by having all the cards face up and then finding the matching pair together, talking about why they are a match (same shape, same color, etc.).

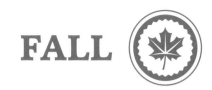

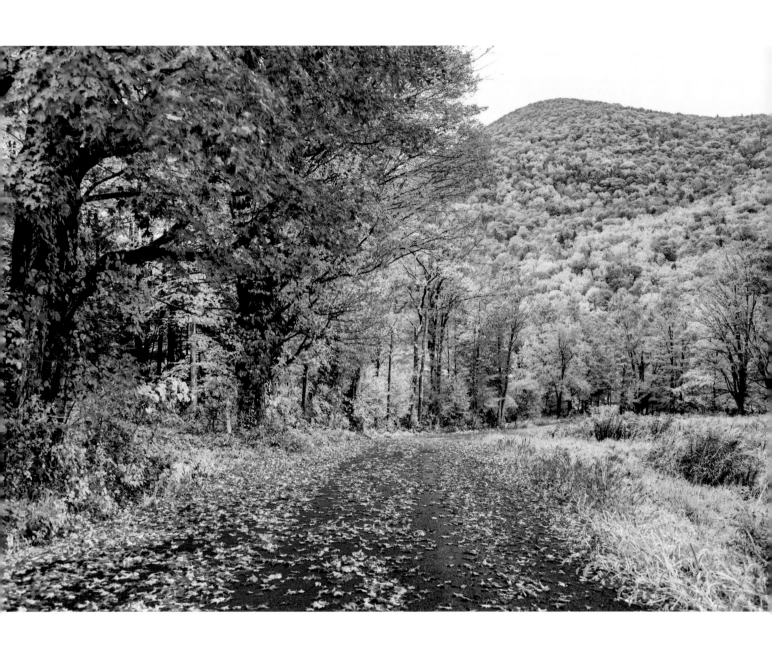

I like to see the leaves change color.

LET'S TALK ABOUT . . .

- When was the first time you voted? What can you tell me about it?

- Where would you vote? What do you remember about voting?

- Did you ever run for office? In school? Or in your community?

- Who was your favorite US president?

- Who was your favorite first lady?

- What campaign slogans do you remember?

- What important political events do you remember?

LET'S TRY . . .

- Talking about different political traditions, such as campaign rallies, slogans, posters, polls, conventions, election-night parties, inaugurations, and so on.

- Looking at books of political cartoons.

- Holding a poll. Decide on a question you would like to ask others to "vote" on, such as a favorite dessert, whether they are left or right handed, or the like. Poll other people together and then tally the results.

- Creating campaign posters together, using poster board, markers, or materials cut out from magazines and newspapers.

- Writing letters to your local representatives on an issue of personal concern.

- Singing patriotic songs, such as "America the Beautiful," "This Land is Your Land," "Happy Days are Here Again," "High Hopes," and others.

- Reading or listening to famous inaugural speeches together (you can find these online).

- Naming different presidents. You can also name different presidential candidates from US history.

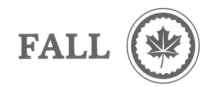

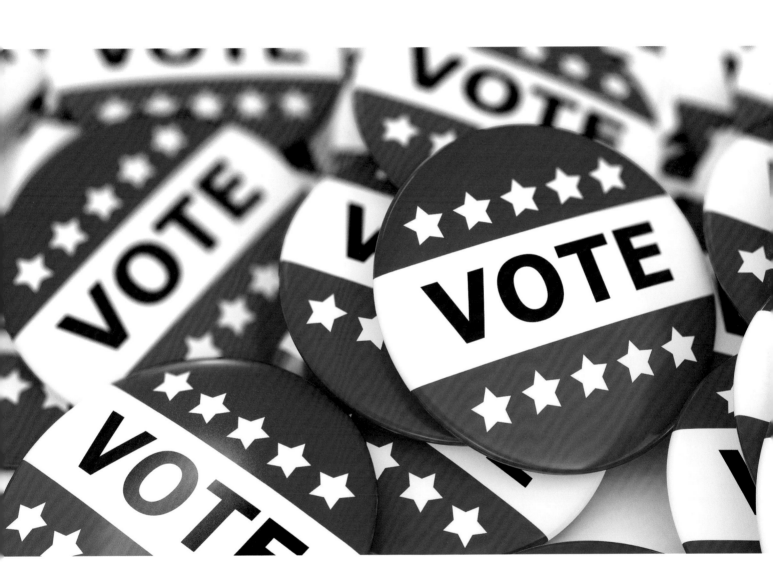

I am proud to vote.

LET'S TALK ABOUT . . .

- Where did you go to school? Can you remember your elementary school? Middle school? High school?

- What was your favorite subject in school? What else did you study?

- Did you have a favorite teacher? What subject did he or she teach?

- How did you get to school? Did you walk, take the bus, or drive?

- What sports did you play in school?

- Did you do any special activities in school, like sing in the chorus, act in school plays, or write for the school newspaper?

- What were your favorite playground games?

- What were your favorite things to eat for lunch at school?

- What would you wear to school? Did you have to wear a school uniform? Were there rules about what you could wear to school?

- How do you think growing up is different today than when you were a child?

LET'S TRY . . .

- Making a school lunch to share together. Assemble a lunch in a paper bag using typical "school" food, such as sandwiches, fruit, chips, drinks, and cookies.

- Decorating a small chalkboard. You will need a small chalkboard in a wooden or other frame, school-themed stickers, colored chalk, string, and a thumbtack (you can find these at a crafts store). Decorate the chalkboard frame with the stickers. Attach the chalk to the board by tying the string to one end of the chalk and using the thumbtack to firmly attach it to the frame. Write or draw together on the chalkboard.

- Sharing school memories about favorite teachers, favorite subjects, school friends, activities, and objects that are used in school.

- Singing favorite school songs together, such as the "Alphabet Song," "School Days," "Be True to Your School," "My Country 'Tis of Thee," and others.

- Creating a collage of school images. You can cut school-related images from magazines or print them from the internet. Cut and glue the images together to a larger piece of paper to create the collage. You can also glue them to an empty, clean cardboard canister or box and use it to hold pens, pencils, rulers, and the like.

- Playing with some favorite schoolyard game materials, such as jacks, jump ropes, footballs, basketballs, bean bags, and other equipment. If able, play the games together.

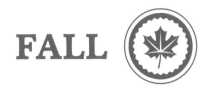

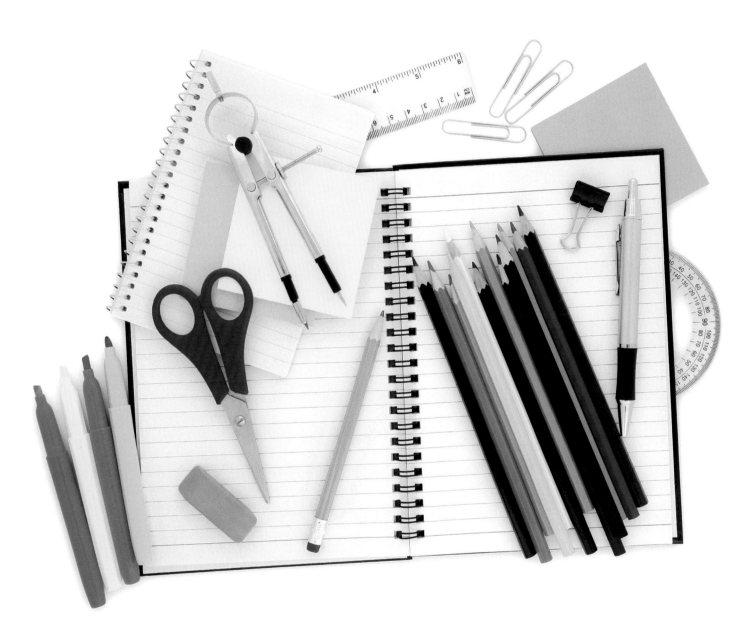

The fall reminds me of school.

LET'S TALK ABOUT . . .

- Did you ever take music or singing lessons?

- Do you play a musical instrument? Which one?

- Were you ever in a band or singing group?

- Who is your favorite singer or musical group?

- What is your favorite kind of music?

- Did you ever see a marching band in a parade or at a sports event? Where did you see one? What do you remember about it?

- Do you have any favorite songs? What are they?

- Where do you listen to music? In the kitchen, in the car, at work?

LET'S TRY . . .

- Naming different musical instruments together.

- Playing some simple instruments, such as a kazoo or recorder, together.

- Listening and singing along together to a playlist of favorite songs (you can create a playlist online).

- Playing marching-band music and having a parade, or "marching" in place, either while standing or seated, in time to the music. You can find marching-band music to listen to online.

- Going to a concert together.

- Listening to and talking about music from different cultures or time periods.

Try to identify the cultural genre of the music (a tango from Spain, a polka from Poland, a western line dance from the United States, etc.).

- Watching a classic musical together.

- Remembering and singing songs that have different words related to fall, such as "autumn," "leaves," and "harvest."

- Creating music together by drumming in rhythm on a table top, clapping hands, or stamping feet. You can keep the rhythms you create together simple or make them more challenging by increasing the length, changing the beat, and so on.

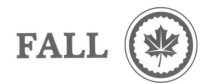

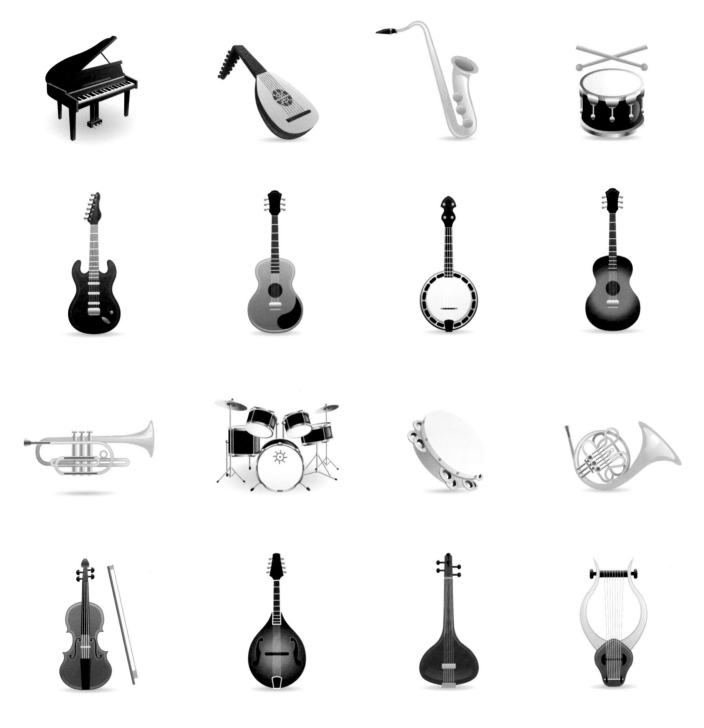

Music makes me happy.

LET'S TALK ABOUT . . .

- Did you ever see a harvest moon? A new moon?

- Did you ever go camping or sleep outside at night? What do you remember about it?

- What do you remember about the first moon landing?

- Let's talk about different astronauts we can remember. Did you have a favorite?

- Have you ever seen a lunar eclipse? A solar eclipse? Can you tell me about it?

- Have you ever dreamed about going to the moon? Why?

- Does your family have traditions that celebrate the harvest or autumn?

LET'S TRY . . .

- Naming the different phases of the moon.

- Talking about the nicknames the full moon has during different months of the year: strawberry moon, hunter's moon, harvest moon, snow moon, and others. (You can learn more about the different moon nicknames online.)

- Singing or listening to songs that refer to the moon together, such as "Harvest Moon" (Neil Young); "Shine On, Harvest Moon" (Rosemary Clooney); and "That's Amore" (Dean Martin).

- Making sugar cookies in the different shapes of the moon's phases.

- Looking together at images of the moon in art throughout history.

- Baking crescent rolls together.

- Taking a trip to the planetarium or natural science museum to see a show or exhibit on space.

- Reading poems about the moon. You can find poems on websites such as www .poets.org or www.poetryfoundation.org.

- Having a harvest festival celebration together. Decorate with traditional harvest decorations, such as small gourds and squashes, Indian corn, and wheat stalks. Serve traditional fall harvest foods, such as corn pudding, apple cider, and sweet potato pie.

- Making a small scarecrow using straw and doll clothing.

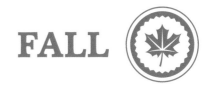

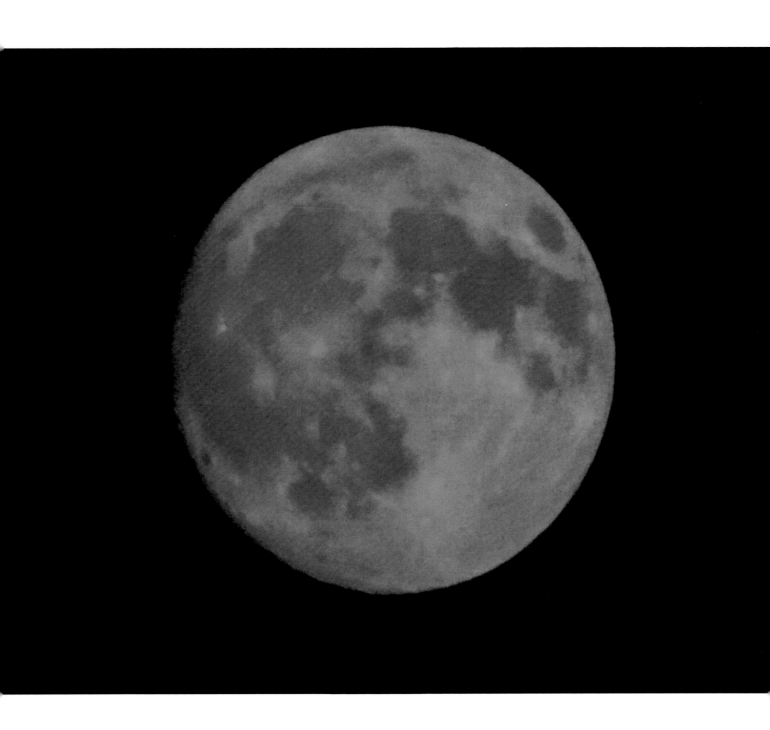

A harvest moon is bright, big, and orange.

LET'S MAKE A MOON AND STARS MOBILE

Create a mobile of the moon and stars together to hang as decor or give as a gift.

You Will Need (you can purchase these items at a crafts store):

- White, yellow, and blue cardstock paper
- Stencils in the shape of the moon, planets, and stars. (You can also cut the shapes out by hand.)
- Hole puncher
- Scissors (safety scissors if needed)
- Nontoxic markers in different colors
- Kitchen twine, kite string, or other string that is easy to tie and handle
- Wire hanger

Instructions

- Use the stencil to trace different moon, star, and planet shapes onto the paper. If desired, decorate the paper shapes with a marker.
- Use the scissors to cut out the shapes.
- Punch holes in the tops of the shapes, where you would like them to hang from, using the hole puncher.
- Next, cut different lengths of the kitchen twine or kite string so that the shapes will hang at different heights.
- Tie the shapes to the hanger, being sure to place the shapes so they will fall at different heights when hung up.
- Hang the mobile and enjoy!

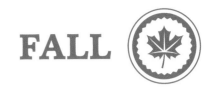

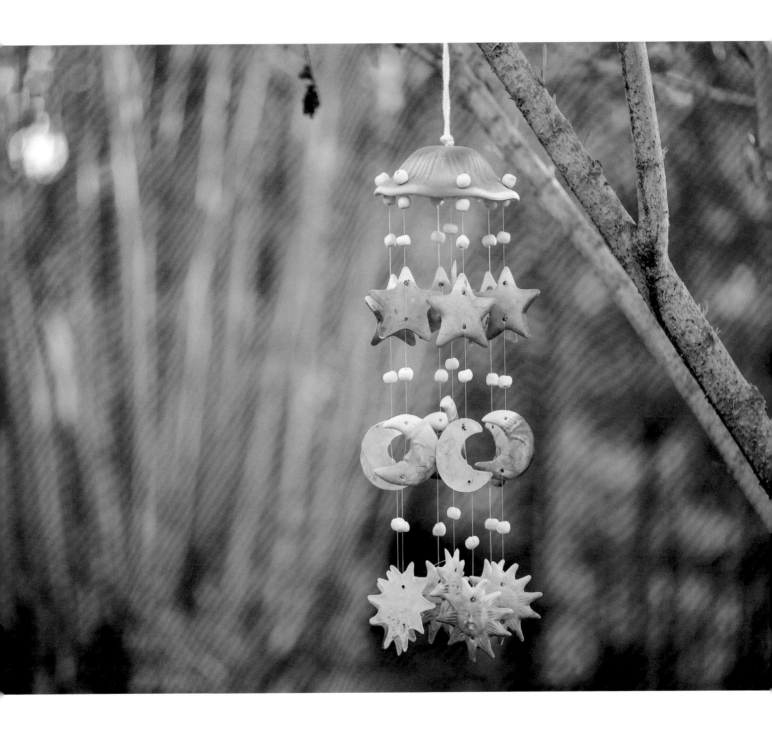

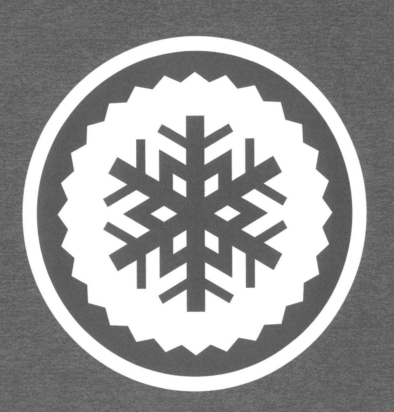

WINTER

LET'S TALK ABOUT . . .

- Did you grow up in a place where there was snow in the winter? What do you remember about snow from when you were younger?

- When did you first see snow?

- Did you ever build a snowman?

- What are some of the things you liked to do in the snow as a child?

- Did you like to go sledding?

- What kinds of games did you play in the snow?

- Do you remember a big snowstorm when you were young?

- What winter sports did you like to do? Did you ski? Ice skate? Play ice hockey?

- What kinds of clothes do you wear to go out in the snow?

- What do you like about winter?

LET'S TRY . . .

- Shaking snow globes to watch the snow fall.

- Making paper snowflakes. Cut snowflake shapes out of paper doilies together. You can use them to decorate the room or windows.

- Making miniature snowmen together. You will need small white foam balls, non-toxic glue, nontoxic markers, and themed stickers (you can find these supplies online or at a crafts store). Stack and glue together 2 or 3 of the balls so that they resemble snowmen. Decorate them using the stickers and markers.

- Singing songs together about snow, such as "Let it Snow," "Frosty the Snowman," or "Jingle Bells."

- Creating "snow" by scraping ice, then feeling its texture and how cold it is.

- Eating a "snow cone" by making a treat out of crushed ice and fruit juice.

- Taking a walk in the snow, talking about how the snow feels, smells, and so on.

- Making a scrapbook using pictures of winter scenes, winter clothing, and other things from wintertime.

- Writing down some favorite wintertime stories from childhood, such as stories about a favorite sledding hill, family winter activities, family recipes, or special holiday memories. Share these stories together with other family members.

- Making a winter-fun memory box. Fill a box with items such as fake snow (cotton balls), pine cones, pine needles, candy canes, gingerbread cookies, cinnamon sticks, jingle bells, and other items.

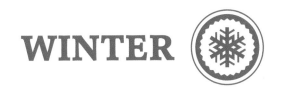

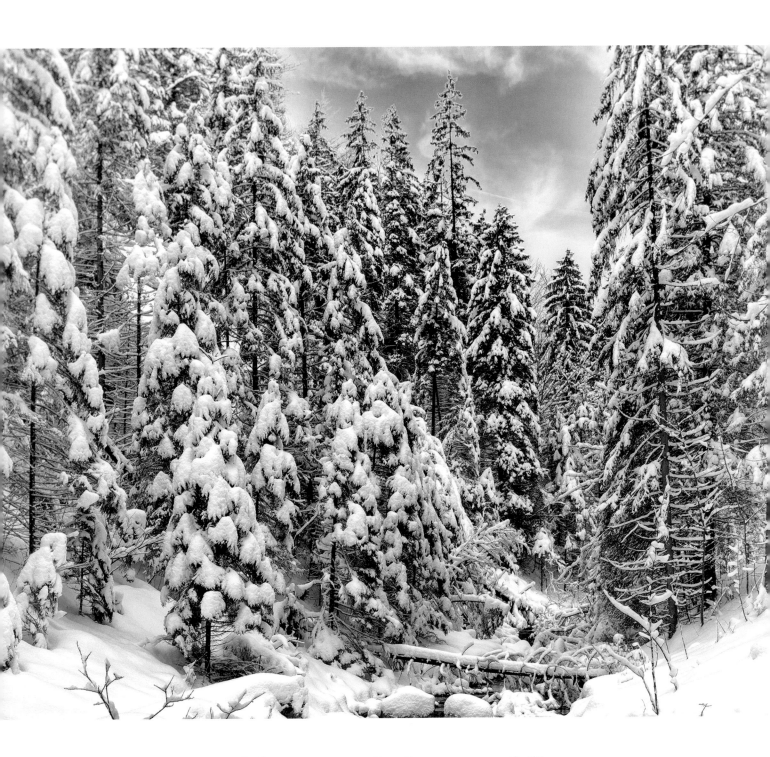

I like to watch the snow fall.

LET'S MAKE A SOCK SNOWMAN

Make a miniature snowman out of common household materials. Use as a winter decoration or gift.

You Will Need (you can purchase these items online or at a crafts store):

- White sock(s)
- Rice
- Scraps of colorful fabric
- Small black beads
- Small orange beads
- Rubber band
- Black fabric marker or paint
- Nontoxic household glue

Instructions

- Open the top of the sock.
- Fill the sock three-quarters full with rice.
- Place a rubber band tightly around the top of the sock, leaving a few inches for the hat.
- To create the hat, fold the lip of the sock over the top of the rubber band.
- Paint the hat with the black paint or marker.
- To add the scarf, take a small strip of the colorful fabric and tie it around the sock (about one-third of the way down from the hat).
- Use the glue and small beads for the snowman's eyes, nose, and mouth. Use the black beads for the coal eyes and mouth and the orange beads for the carrot nose. You could also draw a face using fabric markers.

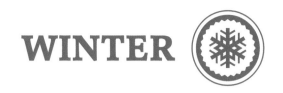

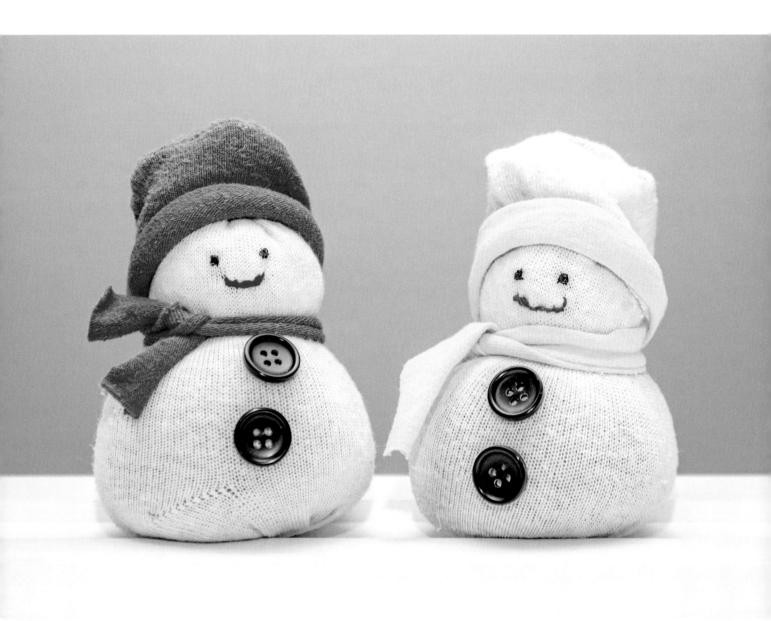

LET'S TALK ABOUT . . .

- Do you have a favorite blanket? What is it made of? What color is it?

- Do you like to sleep in a cold or warm room?

- Did you have a special childhood blanket or blankets that were important to your family?

- Do you like to be wrapped up in a blanket? What does that feel like?

- Did you ever sit under a blanket in front of a fire? Can you tell me about it?

- Did you ever wrap a baby in a blanket? How would you do it?

- Where else could you use a blanket? (At a picnic, in the car, at the beach, while camping, etc.)

- Did you or someone in your family quilt, knit, or crochet?

- Name things that go on the bed (for instance, pillows, blankets, sheets, coverlets, bedspread, throw, duvet, or duvet cover).

- What are some materials blankets are made of?

LET'S TRY . . .

- Touching different kinds of blanket materials, such as wool, cotton, fleece. Let's talk about how they feel to touch and what memories they may bring up.

- Snuggling together under a big blanket or quilt.

- Creating a photo blanket. Use a color printer to make copies of favorite family photographs using iron-on transfer paper. Iron the images onto a large flannel or jersey flat sheet. If desired, you can add labels (names, titles of special events, etc.) to each photograph as you create the iron-on transfers.

- Having an indoor picnic using a blanket on the floor. Serve winter foods, such as warm drinks, soup, chili, and so on.

- Creating a pillow out of old blankets. Stuff a pillowcase with pieces of fabric cut from old blankets. You can glue or sew the open end closed when you are done.

- Purchasing a weighted blanket and trying it together.

- Folding blankets, bed sheets, and towels together.

- Wrapping a baby doll in a blanket.

- Making the bed together.

- Weaving square pot holders using a pot holder weaving loom (you can find pot holder weaving loom kits online or at a local crafts store).

- Cooking and eating pigs in a blanket together (you can find these cocktail treats in the frozen food section of most grocery stores).

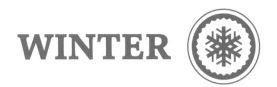

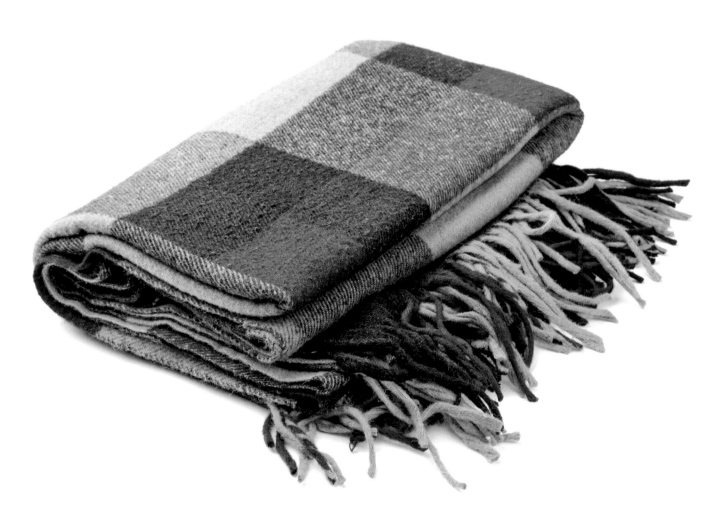

A warm fuzzy blanket on a cold night
makes me feel snug.

LET'S MAKE A NO-SEW THROW BLANKET

This project is one you can easily do together and results in a cozy blanket you both can enjoy. The nature of this activity allows you to space the work across several sessions, and the activity itself can be soothing and relaxing to do.

You Will Need (you can purchase these items online or at a local crafts store):

- Several fleece squares, about 12 × 12 inches, or a no-sew blanket kit with pre-cut squares

- Scissors to cut the fleece

Instructions

- Cut the corners from the fleece squares, about 2 × 2 inches, then cut fringes 1 inch wide and 2 inches deep around the edges of the squares (you will not need to do this if your fleece squares are pre-cut).

- Lay out the squares in the desired pattern.

- Work together to tie the blanket squares to one another, using the fringes.

Photo of the no-sew throw blanket courtesy of www.YourFleece.com.

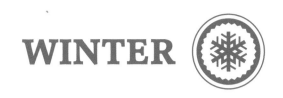

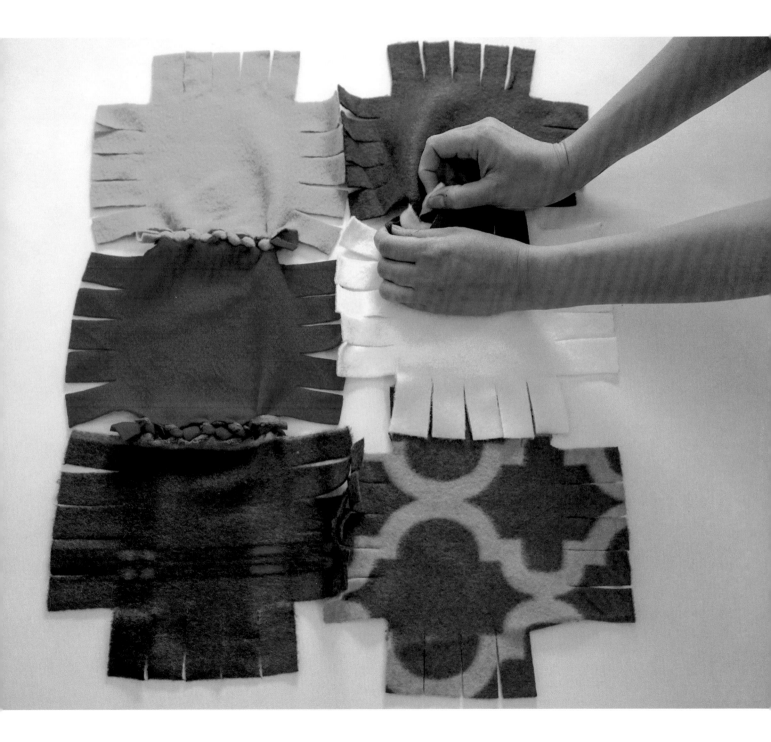

LET'S TALK ABOUT . . .

- What is your favorite kind of cookie?

- Did you ever bake cookies with your mother or grandmother?

- Did you ever bake cookies with children?

- Do you have favorite cookies for the winter holidays?

- Did you keep your cookies in a cookie jar? Can you tell me about it?

- What is your favorite cookie recipe?

- Do you have a special family recipe for cookies? Can you tell me more about it?

- Let's name some different kinds of cookies. (Oatmeal, chocolate chip, animal crackers, sugar, ginger snaps, lemon bars, etc.)

- Let's talk about the different ingredients we use to make cookies. (Flour, sugar, eggs, baking soda, baking powder, nuts, chips, fruits, etc.)

- What did you like to drink with your cookies?

LET'S TRY . . .

- Baking cookies together from premade dough or from scratch.

- Using cookie cutters of different winter-themed shapes to make cookies. Decorate them with white frosting and sugar sprinkles.

- Visiting a local bakery together.

- Wrapping cookies to give as gifts.

- Eating fresh baked cookies with a favorite drink.

- Making a cookie collage using photographs of cookies from magazines.

- Looking at cookbooks with recipes and pictures of different cookies.

- Having a cookie tasting together or with friends. Have several different cookies to taste together. Talk about how they taste, which ones you like and why, and any memories specific cookies may bring.

- "Drawing" with rainbow cookie sprinkles. Place a thin layer of sprinkles in a large-rimmed baking sheet. "Draw" in the sprinkles together using your index fingers to create designs in the sprinkles.

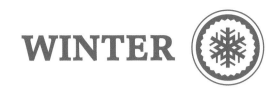

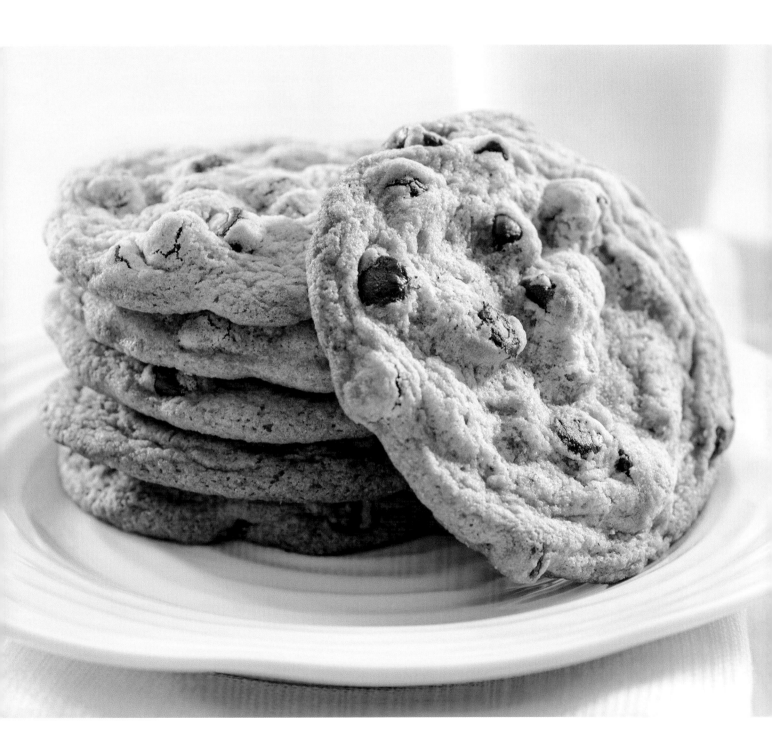

Fresh baked cookies smell delicious.

LET'S TALK ABOUT . . .

- Do you like coffee, tea, hot cider, or hot chocolate?

- What is your favorite flavor of tea?

- Did you ever attend a tea party?

- What do you like to add to your tea or coffee?

- What do you like to eat with your coffee, tea, or hot chocolate?

- What special hot drink was a treat when you were a child?

- Do you like to drink hot chocolate when it is cold outside?

- What memories does hot chocolate remind you of?

- How did you make your hot chocolate? Did you use milk or water? Was it sweet? Spicy? Did you put anything on top?

- Does sipping a hot drink make you feel warm inside?

- Do you like to drink hot drinks in a mug? In a glass? Do you have a favorite mug or glass?

LET'S TRY . . .

- Making hot chocolate together from a mix or from scratch. To make from scratch, melt chocolate and mix with warm milk. Add marshmallows or whipped cream (*optional*).

- Trying hot chocolate recipes from different countries, such as Mexico, France, Spain, or Holland.

- Baking or buying cookies to eat with your hot drink.

- Decorating mugs to use for hot drinks. Mug-making kits are available at most crafts stores.

- Having a tea party. Buy herbal teas and scones and serve tea in pretty tea cups.

- Making finger sandwiches to have with the tea (*see activity*).

- Talking about how tea can be used as an herbal remedy. You can find resources about the health benefits of herbal teas online or at the library.

- Having a tea toss. Line up 3 empty tea tins or mugs. See how many tea bags you can toss in the tin.

- Making hot cider together. Simmer cider with mulling spices, such as cinnamon, cloves, allspice, and ginger. After approximately 15–20 minutes, strain cider and serve in mugs.

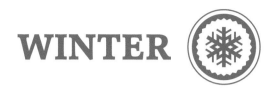

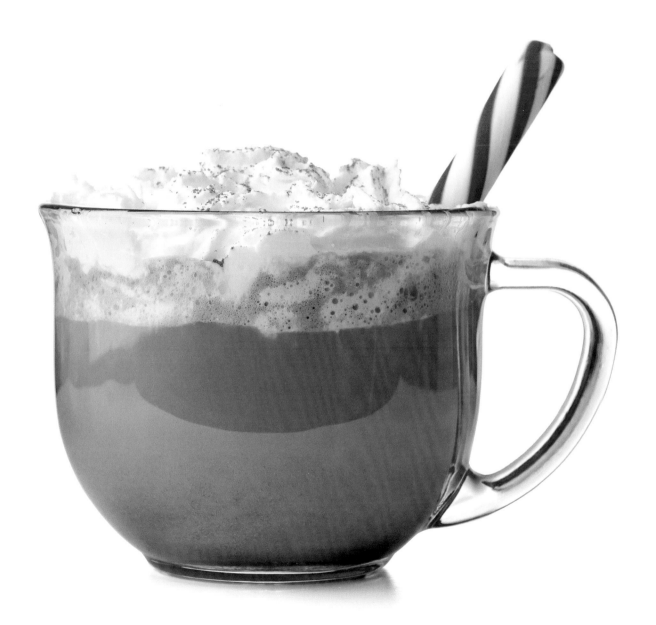

Hot drinks warm me up on a cold winter day.

LET'S MAKE TEA SANDWICHES

This simple activity is a wonderful way to share something special on a cold wintry afternoon.

You Will Need:

- White, whole wheat, or other favorite breads, thinly sliced
- Tea sandwich ingredients (*see below*)
- Knives for spreading and cutting the sandwiches

Instructions

- Choose your favorite tea sandwiches from the recipe ideas below.
- Assemble the sandwiches according to the directions.
- Cut the crust off of the sandwiches. Next, cut the sandwiches into quarters or lengthwise into "fingers."
- Place sandwiches on a tray or plate to share, along with a selection of hot teas.

Tea Sandwiches: Suggested Recipes

Butter, Cucumber, and Radish Sandwiches
Spread softened butter on 2 slices of your bread of choice. Make sandwich using thinly sliced rounds of cucumber and radishes. Salt and pepper to taste. Trim the crusts and cut into pieces.

Tomato-Cheddar Sandwiches
Spread Dijonnaise mustard on 2 slices of your bread of choice. Make sandwich using sliced tomato, aged cheddar cheese, and watercress or arugula. Trim the crusts and cut into pieces.

Ham, Brie, and Apple Sandwiches
Spread Dijon mustard on 2 slices of your bread of choice. Fill with deli ham, sliced brie cheese, and sliced green apple. Trim the crusts and cut into pieces.

Egg Salad Sandwiches
Mix 3 chopped hard-boiled eggs with ¼ cup mayonnaise. Salt and pepper to taste. Spread additional mayonnaise on 2 slices of your bread of choice. Fill sandwich with the egg salad. Trim the crusts and cut into pieces.

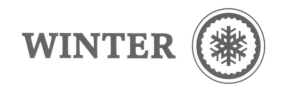

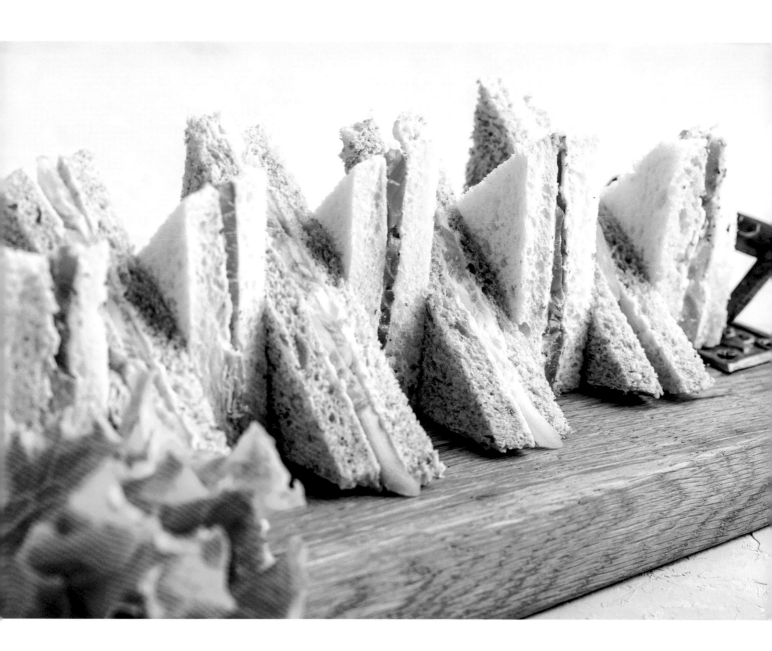

LET'S TALK ABOUT . . .

- Did you ever watch the Winter Olympics? Which Olympics do you remember?

- Can you think of some sports played in the Winter Olympics?

- Let's name some countries that compete in the Olympics.

- Let's name countries that have hosted the Winter Olympics.

- What is your favorite winter sport to watch?

- Let's name some famous Winter Olympians.

- Did you take part in a winter sport, such as skiing, ice hockey, or skating? Can you tell me about it?

- Did you ever go sledding? What do you remember about it?

- What does it feel like when you are outside in winter?

- What do you wear to play a sport outside in the winter?

LET'S TRY . . .

- Watching people ice skating at an outdoor lake or indoor skating rink.

- Going to see an ice hockey game.

- Watching videos of past Winter Olympics, including videos of the opening ceremonies and different events (you can find videos online).

- Making Olympic medals and hanging them up for decoration or giving them as gifts.

- Listening to and singing different national anthems (you can find videos and lyrics for different national anthems online).

- Playing Olympic ring toss (*see activity*).

- Identifying different national flags (you can find images online).

- Watching an old movie about winter sports, such as *Sun Valley Serenade, Ice Castles, The Cutting Edge, Downhill Racer, Miracle on Ice, Slap Shot,* or *The Mighty Ducks.*

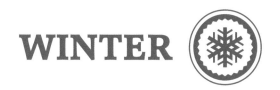

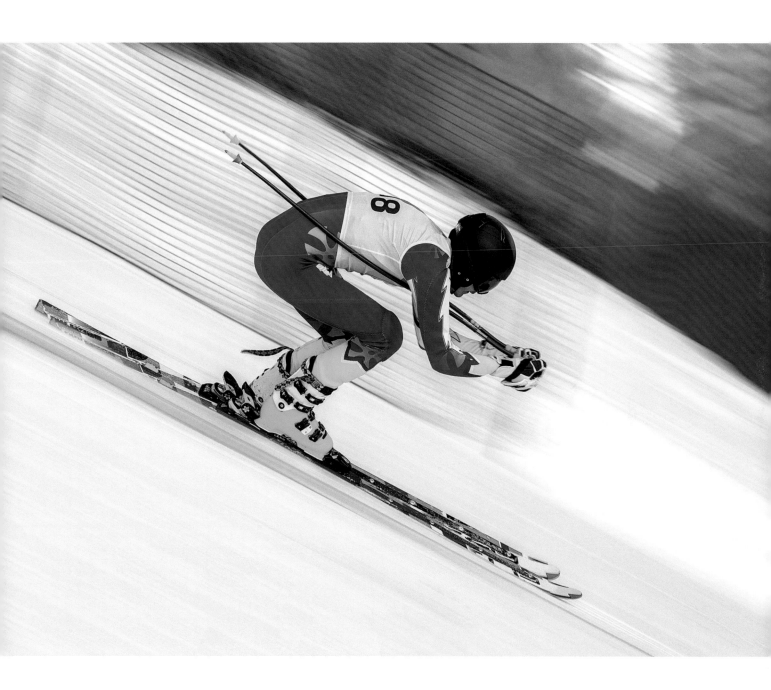

It is exciting to watch the Winter Olympics on TV.

LET'S MAKE AN OLYMPIC RING TOSS

This is a fun way to bring a bit of the Olympic spirit to your day!

You Will Need (you can purchase these items online or at a local crafts store):

- 5 embroidery rings
- 2-liter plastic bottle, filled with liquid or sand (so that it will not easily be knocked over)
- Colored duct tape, including the colors of the Olympic rings (black, red, green, blue, and yellow)

Instructions

- Decorate your 2-liter bottle with assorted duct tape in the colors of the Olympic rings.
- Next, wrap each of your embroidery hoops in duct tape in one of the Olympic ring colors (one each in black, red, green, blue, and yellow).
- Play by tossing the "Olympic rings" and seeing who can land the most rings on the bottle target.

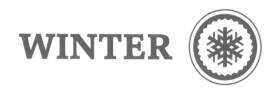

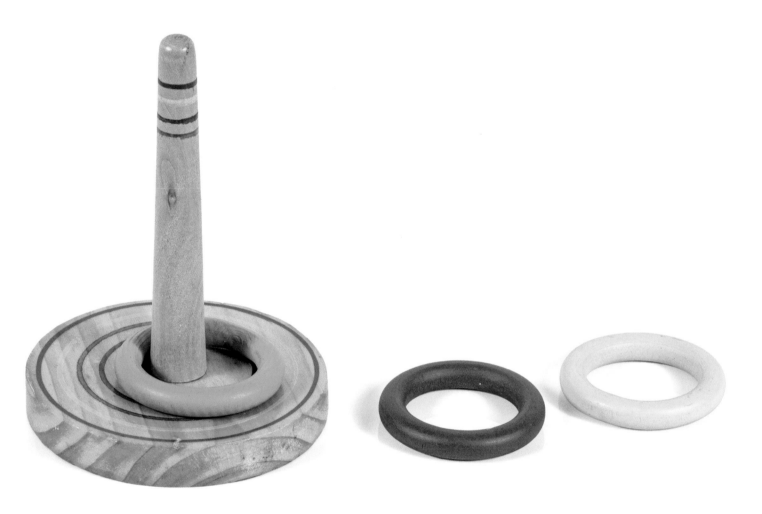

LET'S TALK ABOUT . . .

▸ Can you name different kinds of holiday lights? (Christmas string lights and luminarias, Chanukah candles, Kwanzaa kinara, etc.)

▸ What different holidays does your family celebrate throughout the year?

▸ What is your favorite holiday? Why is it your favorite?

▸ Let's talk about some special foods we eat at the holidays.

▸ What kinds of lights do you use for the holidays (stringed lights, candles, etc.)? Where do you put them?

▸ Does your family have special holiday traditions? What are they?

▸ Do you have a favorite holiday dish? What is it? How is it made?

▸ What are some of your favorite holiday memories from when you were a child?

▸ Do you have a favorite holiday movie or play? Can you tell me about it?

▸ Can you name some of your favorite holiday gifts that you have gotten?

LET'S TRY . . .

▸ Taking a walk or drive through the neighborhood or to a local shopping area to look at the different holiday lights.

▸ Making holiday cards for others in need together. You can send the cards to soldiers serving in the armed forces, hospital patients, isolated elderly, and so on. Find where to send cards in your community by checking with local hospitals, food pantries, or other organizations.

▸ Playing holiday-card concentration. You will need 10–12 holiday cards. Make sure that you have 5–6 pairs of cards with matching images (two dreidels, two Christmas trees, etc.). Trim the cards so that they are all the same size and shape, leaving the pictures or designs in the center intact. To play, turn all the cards face down, then work together turning over two cards at a time until you find a match. Leave the matched cards face up.

▸ Filling a bowl with holiday-themed items and exploring them together. Include, for example, items such as evergreen cuttings, holiday decorations, candles, small strings of holiday lights, pine cones, and a snow globe.

▸ Smelling different scents of the holidays together. Purchase aromatherapy oils or items at the grocery store scented with evergreen, pine, peppermint, cinnamon, and the like. Smell the scents one at a time, talking about what memories they bring up, which ones you like best, and so on.

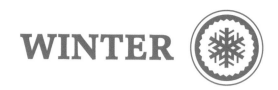

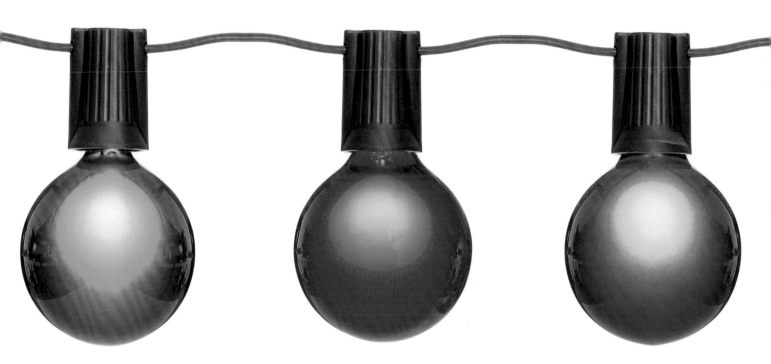

Lights make the holidays festive and bright.

LET'S MAKE BEESWAX CANDLES

Make these lovely candles together to give as holiday gifts for family or friends.

You Will Need (you can purchase these items online or at a local crafts store):

- 3–4 sheets of honeycomb beeswax
- Candlewick string
- Wax paper
- Scissors
- Hair blow-dryer
- Masking tape

Instructions

- Place a sheet of wax paper a little longer than the honeycomb beeswax sheet on a flat surface with the narrow end toward your loved one. Tape down the ends of the wax paper to hold it in place.

- Next, place a sheet of beeswax on top of the wax paper, with the narrow end toward your loved one.

- Use the blow-dryer to slightly warm the wax so that it will not be brittle and break as you roll it (but be careful not to melt it).

- Cut a piece of candlewick about 2 inches longer than the narrow end of the bees-wax sheet. Place the wick at the narrow end of your beeswax sheet closest to your loved one.

- Begin to roll the candle, helping your loved one roll the beeswax sheet slowly and carefully around the wick.

- When done, gently lift the candle off the wax paper and crimp the edge of the beeswax sheet slightly into the body of the candle.

- If desired, you may trim the piece of wick off the "bottom" end of the candle.

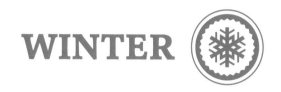

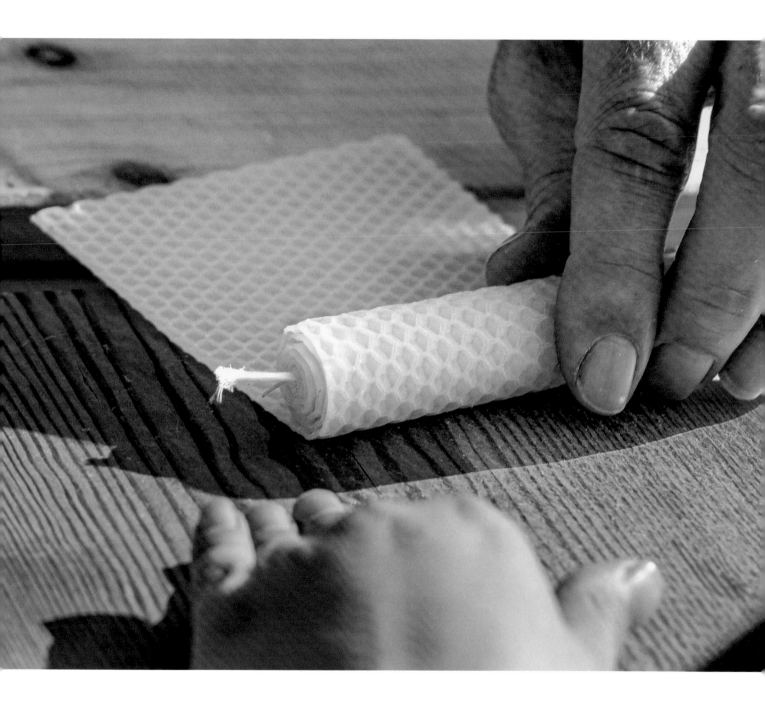

LET'S TALK ABOUT . . .

- What is your favorite country to visit?

- Where did you go on your honeymoon?

- What was your favorite place to take a family vacation?

- If you could visit any country which one would it be?

- Do you like to travel by plane, car, or boat? Which is your favorite?

- Did you ever get lost while traveling? What did you do?

- Do you like to go to places in the city or in the countryside?

- What was a favorite city you stayed in?

- What items do you need to pack when you travel?

LET'S TRY . . .

- Going to the local library to check out travel books or videos.

- Creating a meal themed around a specific country, such as France or Mexico.

- Talking about the country your family came from and the traditions your family brought from that country.

- Going to a concert or listening to music from a specific country.

- Visiting a neighborhood or restaurant known for its ties to a specific culture.

- Playing "What's in the Bag?" Fill a small travel bag with different travel items, such as travel-sized toiletries, luggage tags, an eye mask, ear plugs, and so on. Take turns feeling an item in the bag and guessing what it is. Remove each item when it is guessed correctly.

- Making a travel collage using pictures from travel magazines.

- Studying maps together using an atlas or road maps.

- Planning and taking a local road trip together to visit historical or noted sites.

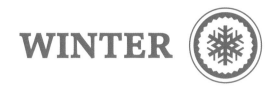

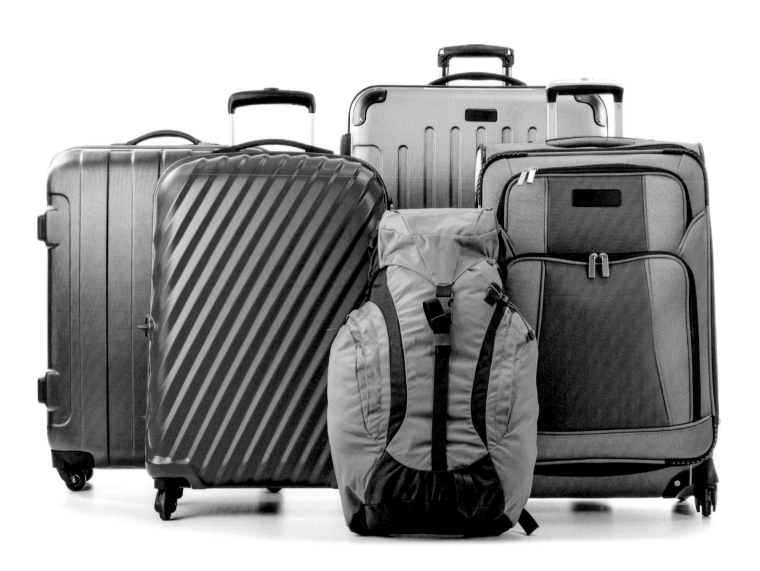

I like to visit different places.

LET'S TALK ABOUT . . .

- What is your favorite soup? What do you like about it?

- Did your family have a special soup for the holidays? What was it?

- Did you ever eat cold soup? Which one did you eat?

- Do you like to eat soup in a bowl or a mug? Why?

- Let's name different kinds of soup together.

- What kinds of things do you eat with soup? (Crackers, bread, tortilla chips, grilled cheese, croutons, etc.)

- What is the strangest soup you ever ate?

LET'S TRY . . .

- Making a favorite soup together from scratch or using a boxed soup.

- Having soups from around the world together. Try soup recipes from different countries, adding to the experience with utensils, bowls, and decor from that culture.

- Collecting and donating cans of soup to a food pantry together.

- Creating bean art jars. Take different dried beans and legumes of different shapes and colors (black beans, chickpeas, lentils, etc.). Fill glass jars with the beans and legumes, alternating to create different layers of varying colors and shapes. When filled, place the lid on the jar and finish with a ribbon or by gluing on beans.

- Reading stories together from *Chicken Soup for the Soul.*

- Visiting a grocery store and looking through all the different kinds of soup on sale.

- Decorating soup mugs or bowls together. Visit a pottery-painting shop or purchase a kit to make them online.

- Baking bread together to have with the soup. Buy frozen loaves at the grocery store or bake from scratch.

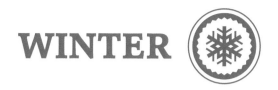

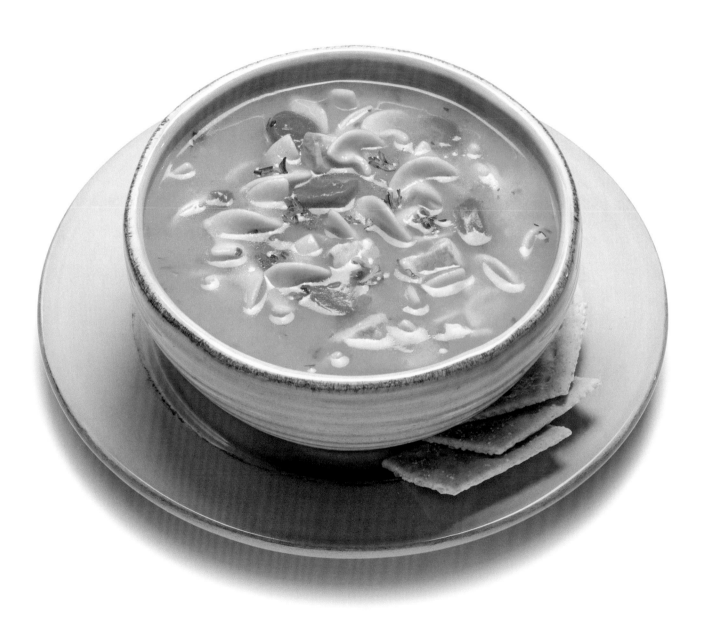

Soup warms me up when it is cold outside.

LET'S MAKE MINESTRONE SOUP

Make this simple, delicious vegetable soup to share together and with friends.

You Will Need:

- 2 tablespoons olive oil
- 2 cloves garlic, peeled and chopped
- 1 large yellow onion, peeled and chopped
- 28 oz can crushed tomatoes
- 8 oz can chopped tomatoes
- 3 medium carrots, peeled and diced
- 2 stalks celery, chopped
- 8 oz can cannellini beans
- 8 oz can kidney beans
- 2–3 cups fresh or frozen green beans, trimmed and cut into ½ inch pieces
- 1 teaspoon dried Italian seasoning
- Salt and pepper to taste
- 10–12 cups of water
- 1 cup orzo or other small pasta, cooked
- Grated parmesan cheese or pesto to garnish before serving (*optional*)

Instructions

- Heat the olive oil in a large pot over medium-high heat.
- Add the onion and cook until translucent, about 4 minutes.
- Add the garlic. After about 30 seconds, add the celery and carrots. Cook until softened, about 5 minutes.
- Stir in the green beans, Italian seasoning, salt, and pepper. Cook another 3–5 minutes.
- Add the diced and crushed tomatoes and water to the pot. Bring to a boil.
- Reduce the heat to medium-low heat and simmer 10 minutes more.
- Stir in the kidney and cannellini beans and cook about 10 minutes.
- Add cooked pasta and simmer for another 5 minutes until pasta is warmed through.
- Ladle soup into bowls. If desired, top with grated parmesan cheese or a teaspoon of pesto before serving.

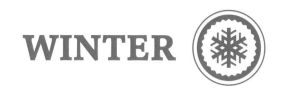

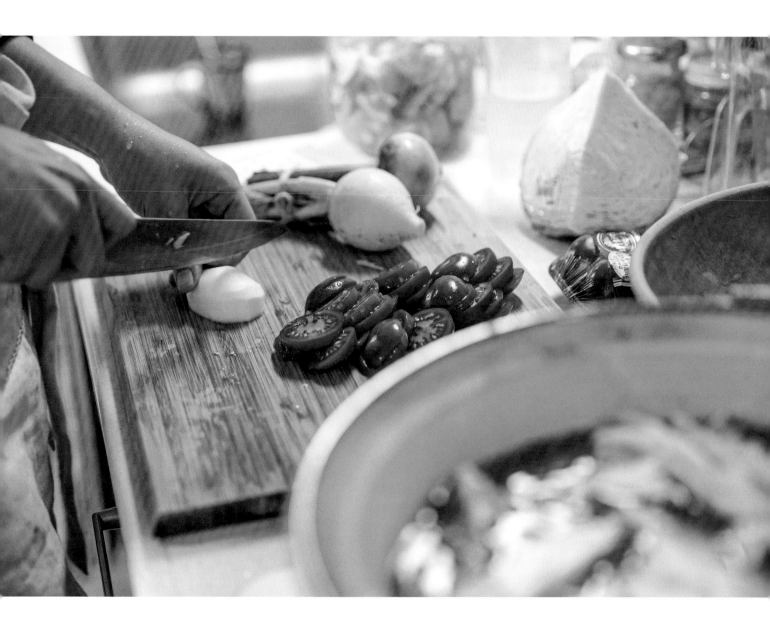

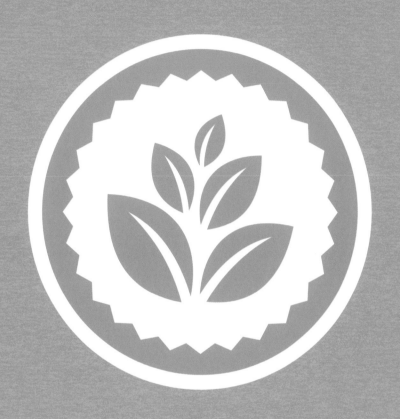

SPRING

- Do you remember a very windy day in spring?

- Did you hang your laundry out to dry on windy days? Where was your clothesline? Let's talk about what laundry you would put on the clothesline.

- Do you like to fly a kite on a windy day? Do you have a favorite spot for flying a kite? Who taught you to fly a kite, can you tell me about that? Did you ever teach someone to fly a kite?

- Do you like to listen to wind chimes?

- What different sounds does the wind make?

- Have you ever been in a windstorm? Like a twister, hurricane, or sandstorm?

LET'S TRY . . .

- Making a simple kite out of brown paper, craft sticks, fabric strips, and string. You can decorate the kite with stickers and markers. (You can find these supplies at a crafts store or online.)

- Creating a wind indicator out of some long fabric strips and a stick. You can mount the wind indicator outside a window and use it to see when the wind is blowing.

- Listening to wind chimes. Try wind chimes of different sizes, shapes, and materials. Talk about their different sounds.

- Making wind chimes by tying shells onto a wire loop. You will need shells with holes drilled at the top, string, and a wire loop. (You can find these supplies at a crafts store.)

- Blowing across the top of an open bottle and listening to the sound. You can fill bottles with different amounts of water and try "playing" simple songs such as "Jack and Jill" and "Row, Row, Row Your Boat" by blowing on the bottles.

- Taking a walk together on a windy spring day.

- Playing a parachute game. Take a sheet, grab the sides, and move it up and down to create wind.

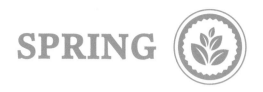

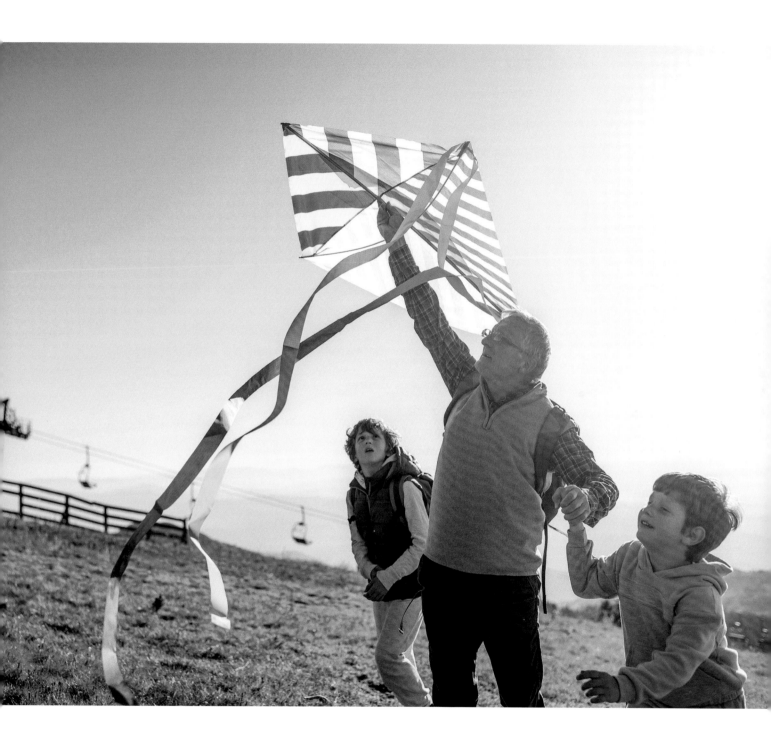

I like feeling the wind blow on spring days.

LET'S TALK ABOUT . . .

- Did you ever take dancing lessons?

- What type of dancing do you like to do?

- Do you like slow dancing or fast dancing?

- Did you ever square or line dance?

- What folk dances do you know?

- What dances were popular when you were in high school?

- Can you name some different dance steps?

- Do you like to watch dancing? Do you have some favorite dance shows?

- Can you name some famous ballets?

- Can you name some famous dancers?

- Did you ever go to prom? What do you remember about it?

LET'S TRY . . .

- Dancing to your favorite songs together, either while standing or seated.

- Playing and naming different dance music. (Salsa, swing, polka, waltz, line, Irish jig, etc.)

- Matching dances to their country or region of origin. For example: tango (Argentina), lion dance (China), polka (Czech Republic or Poland), cancan (France), tarantella (Italy), flamenco (Spain), or waltz (Austria).

- Going to see a dance recital in your community.

- Watching famous dance movies, such as *Singin' in the Rain, Grease, Dirty Dancing, Footloose, The Turning Point*, or movies with famous dancers, such as Gene Kelly, Fred Astaire, Ginger Rogers, Shirley Temple.

- Having a "senior"-prom date, including dressing up, wearing a corsage, having dinner, and dancing. Consider holding a "senior" prom in your community, inviting families or intergenerational guests to participate.

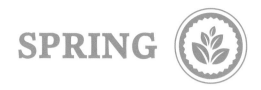

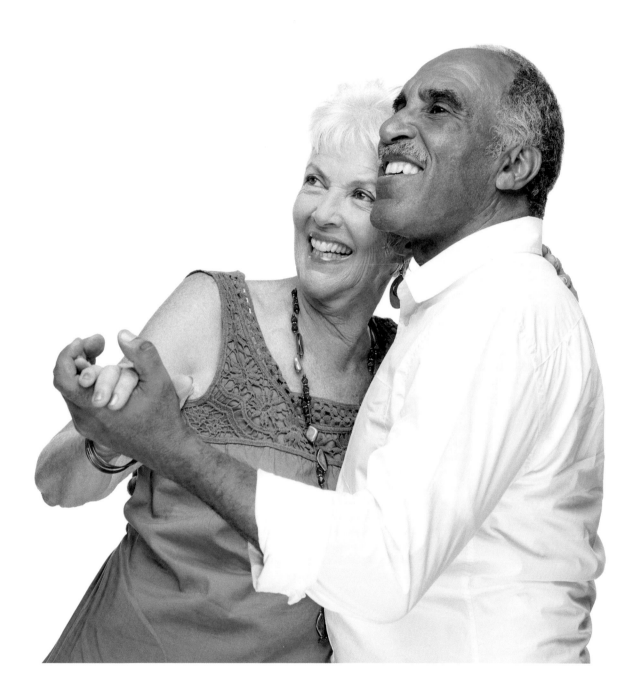

Dancing makes me feel young at heart.

LET'S TALK ABOUT . . .

- Do you have any favorite flowers? What are they?

- Have you ever visited a special flower garden? Where?

- Did you have a flower garden when you were a child? What do you remember about it?

- Butterflies are a special part of a flower garden. Can you name different kinds of butterflies? Do you have a favorite butterfly?

- What colors do you like to see in a garden?

- Which flowers' scents do you like best? (For instance, rose, lavender, lily of the valley, or jasmine.)

- Did you have flowers at your wedding? What kinds of flowers did you have?

- Name different types of spring flowers. (Azaleas, cherry blossoms, hyacinths, snap dragons, tulips, dahlias, irises, etc.)

LET'S TRY . . .

- Planting spring bulbs you can enjoy either in an outdoor garden or in a pot. You can find advice on planting bulbs and planting materials online or at your local garden center.

- Volunteering at a local flower garden for a few hours a week.

- Visiting a local garden or park together, talking about the different flowers and plantings.

- Making a flower scrapbook. Cut out photographs of different flowers and glue them in a scrapbook. You can also add other flower-themed items, such as seed packets, pictures of gardening tools, and the like.

- Singing familiar songs about flowers, such as "Daisy Bell (Bicycle Built for Two)," "Tip Toe through the Tulips," or "Roses are Red."

- Arranging a flower bouquet in a vase.

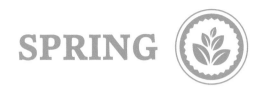

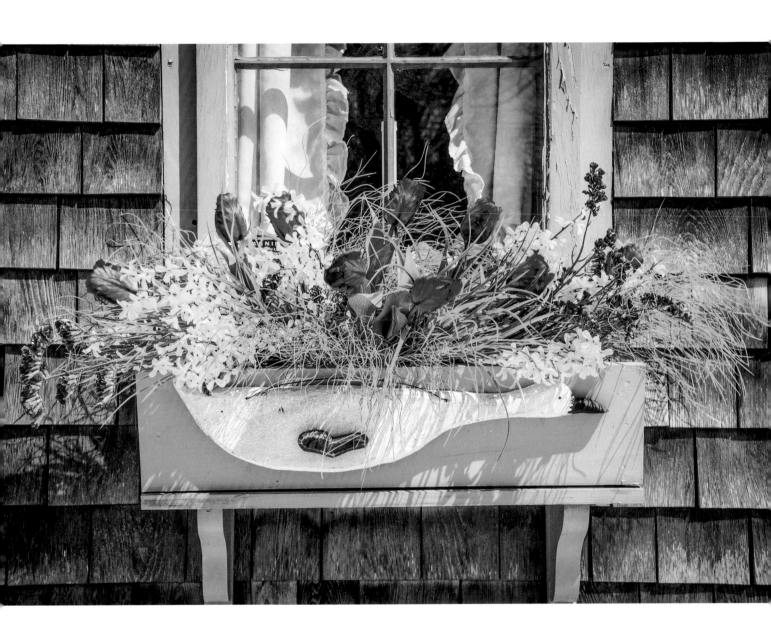

Spring flowers are lovely to see and smell.

Make scented sachets out of dried flowers to use in a clothing drawer or closet or to give as gifts.

You Will Need (you can purchase these items online or at a crafts store):

- Dried flower mix
- Floral scented oils
- Small sachet bags
- Thin ribbon
- Large mixing bowl
- Wooden mixing spoon

Instructions

- Place the dried flower mix in the mixing bowl.
- Smell the different scented oils together, talking about each one. Choose one or a combination of them for the sachets.
- Sprinkle the dried flower mix with a few drops of the scented oil(s) and stir gently.
- Open one of the sachet bags. Fill it with the mix to 2 inches below the top of the bag. Close the bag using the drawstrings provided. Add a decorative piece of ribbon and/or bow.

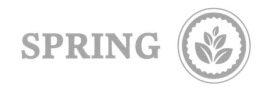

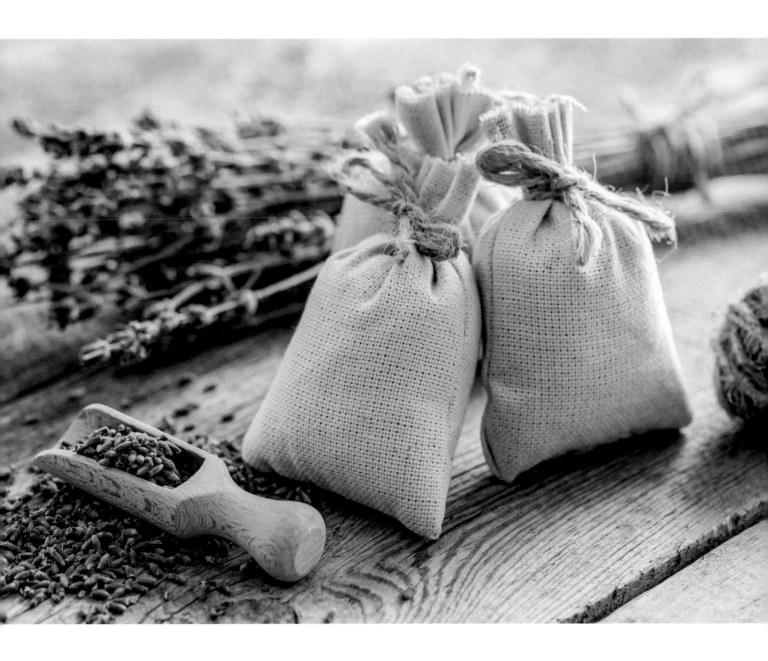

LET'S TALK ABOUT . . .

- What are the different sounds that birds make?

- Can you name some types of birds? Where would you find that kind of bird? By water, in a garden, or in the woods? (Wrens, owls, ducks, robins, chickens, bluebirds, blackbirds, seagulls, cardinals, ostriches, blue jays, doves, humming-birds, etc.)

- What is your favorite kind of bird?

- Did you ever have a pet bird? What kind? What was its name?

- What does the sound of birds singing in the spring make you think of?

- Did you ever see a bird's nest? What did you see inside?

LET'S TRY . . .

- Making a bird feeder and hanging it outside the window. (You can get bird-feeder kits online or at a crafts store.)

- Stringing together pretzels or cereal, such as Cheerios, and hanging the string outside the window for the birds to eat.

- Building a birdbath. Put a large bowl of water on a chair or short pillar outside, where it will be visible from the window. Watch the birds use it as a birdbath.

- Touching different feathers and talking about how they feel on our hands, faces, or necks. (You can purchase feathers online or at a crafts store.)

- Taking a walk in the neighborhood or local park and looking and listening for different types of birds.

- Visiting a local aviary or zoo.

- Listening to recorded birdcalls online or on tape.

- Looking at pictures in a bird-watching handbook.

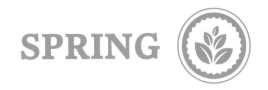

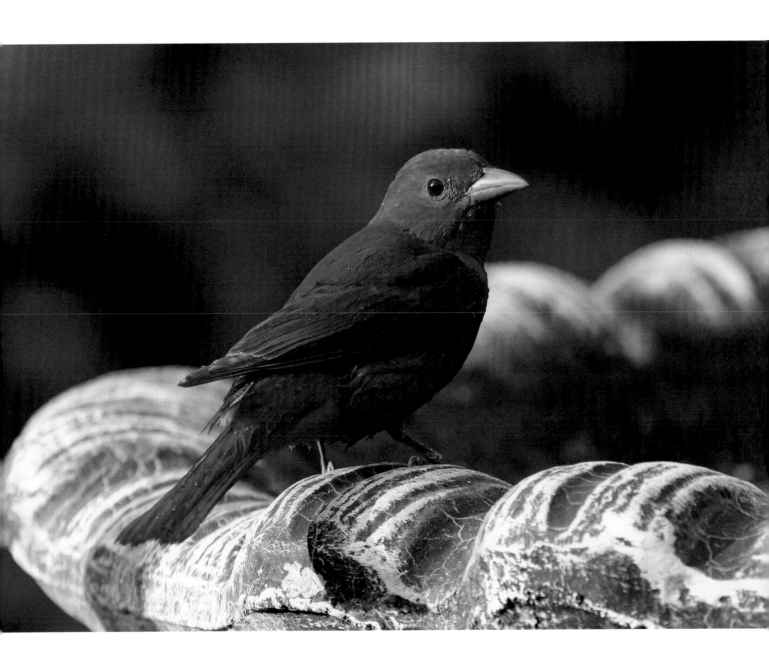

Hearing the birds on a spring morning
makes me happy.

LET'S TALK ABOUT . . .

- Tell me about the different homes you have lived in.

- Did you ever rent a home or apartment? Did you own a home or apartment?

- What kinds of home-improvement projects did you do? Did you enjoy them?

- What chores did you do for spring-cleaning?

- What were some of the cleaning products you used?

- What chores did you do as a child?

- Do you have any favorite cleaning tips?

- What tools did you have in your toolkit? (Hammer, screwdriver, wrench, etc.)

- What tools did you use the most?

LET'S TRY . . .

- Looking at pictures of different homes in home magazines or books.

- Watching home-improvement shows together and talking about the projects.

- Cleaning together. Dust, vacuum, reorganize drawers or closets.

- Putting together a toolkit with different tools commonly used in a household. Talk about each of the tools, how they are used and what projects you can use them for.

- Putting together a basket with common household cleaning supplies. Talk about and use the different supplies as you are able. For safety, empty containers, rinse clean, and refill with nontoxic materials (that is, water with a few drops of essential oils, such as pine, for scent).

- Building a simple birdhouse. You can purchase a birdhouse kit online or from a pet or garden center. Work together to assemble and decorate the birdhouse.

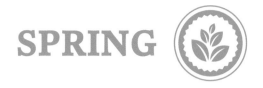

SPRING

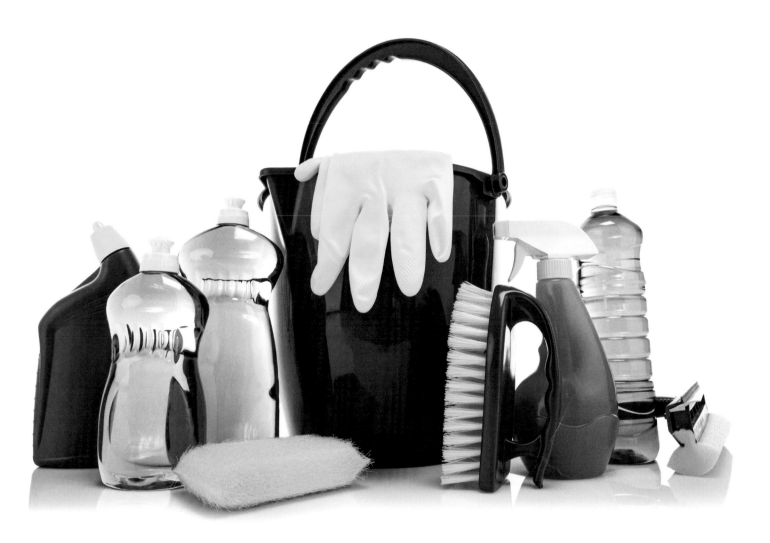

Spring is a good time for home-improvement projects.

LET'S TALK ABOUT . . .

- Name some things to do on a rainy day.

- Did you ever play games in the rain as a child? What were they?

- Have you ever been caught in a big rainstorm? What was it like?

- What are some things that happen when it rains? (For example, the gutters bring water down from the roof, the sidewalks form puddles, and the flowers get watered.)

- What animals live in water? (Frogs, fish, snakes, etc.)

- What colors do you see in a rainbow after it rains? Did you ever see a rainbow?

- What do you need to wear when you go out in the rain?

LET'S TRY . . .

- Taking a walk together in the rain. (Wait for a day when the rain is gentle or misting.) Talk about the different smells and sights.

- Making a rainy-day jar. Take an empty glass or plastic container and put it outside to collect the rain. Use the rain you collect to experience the rain more closely by smelling, touching, and looking at the collected rain together. Use the rain you collected to water the plants. (Do not drink the rainwater or use with food.)

- Talking about times in history when rainstorms played a major part in current events, such as the 1930s Dust Bowl, the 1937 Ohio River flood, Hurricane Katrina, and others. Look at news stories and photographs of those events.

- Singing songs about the rain, such as "Rain, Rain Go Away," "Singin' in the Rain," "Raindrops Keep Falling on My Head," and "Who'll Stop the Rain."

- Listening to different recordings of rain sounds.

- Finding famous movie scenes that include rain, such as *Singin' in the Rain*, *Butch Cassidy and the Sundance Kid*, and *Breakfast at Tiffany's*.

- Talking about rain-related garments and accessories, such as rain hats, rain boots, ponchos, and umbrellas. Show pictures of the items or use the actual garments.

- Making a rainbow. Buy a small prism at a crafts store. Use the sunlight in the room to make a rainbow.

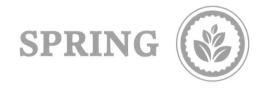

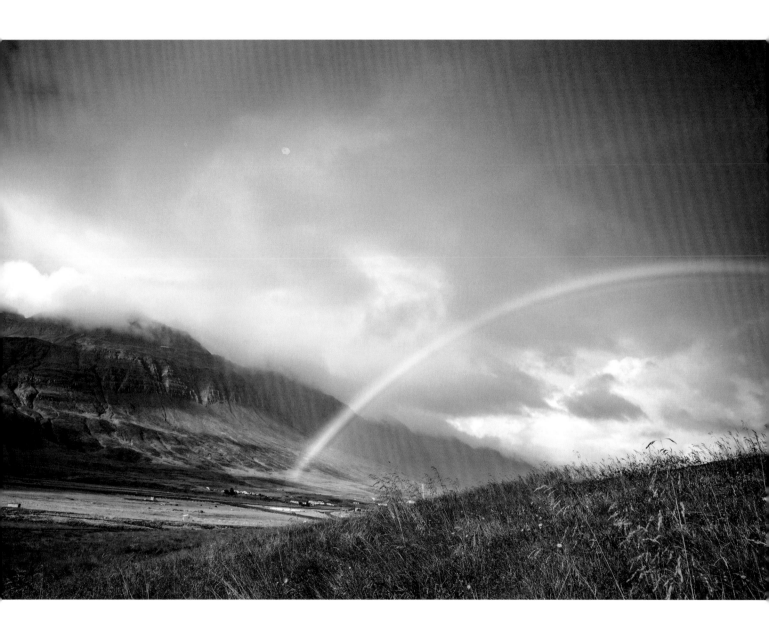

Rain makes the air smell fresh and clean.

LET'S TALK ABOUT . . .

▸ Did you ever spend time with a pet?

▸ Did you ever own a pet? What kind of pet did you have? What was your pet's name?

▸ Did you ever own a more unusual pet, such as a reptile, rabbit, or horse?

▸ What kinds of tricks did you teach your pet?

▸ What color was your pet?

▸ What do you think makes a better pet: a cat or a dog?

▸ Did you have a favorite pet? Tell me more about that pet.

▸ Where did your pet sleep?

▸ What did your pet eat?

▸ Do you enjoy watching shows about dogs or cats on TV?

▸ Can you tell me any funny stories about your pet?

LET'S TRY . . .

▸ Visiting a local pet store, zoo, horse barn, or farm.

▸ Finding a local pet-therapy group to bring a pet to you. Check out this website to find a group in your area: http://www.akc.org /events/title-recognition-program/therapy /organizations/.

▸ Singing songs about pets, such as "How Much is That Doggie in the Window," "Old Shep" or "Hound Dog" (Elvis Presley), "A Horse with No Name" (America), and "Nashville Cats" (The Lovin' Spoonful).

▸ Making homemade dog biscuits and bringing them to a local shelter (*see activity*).

▸ Naming some famous cats and dogs (Lassie, Rin Tin Tin, Garfield, Cat in the Hat, Felix, etc.).

▸ Naming different breeds of dogs and cats.

▸ Looking at pictures of different pet breeds.

▸ Playing a bone-toss game. Get a large dog bowl and 3 different size biscuits. Place the bowl on a table or floor and toss the biscuits in the bowl.

▸ Making a cat or dog collage using old magazines.

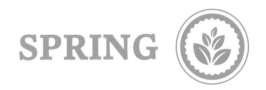

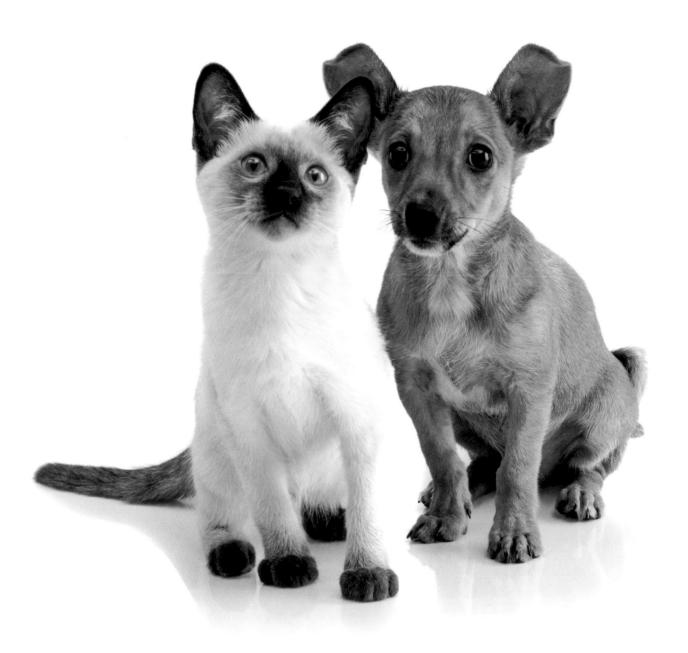

Spending time with a pet makes me feel good.

LET'S MAKE DOG BISCUITS

Bake dog biscuits together to share with pet-owning friends or donate to a local pet shelter.

You Will Need:

- 2 cups flour
- ½ cup peanut butter
- 2 eggs
- ¼ cup of water

- Large mixing bowl
- Rolling pin
- Cookie cutters
- Cookie sheet

Instructions

- Preheat the oven to 350 degrees
- Mix together peanut butter, eggs, and flour in large bowl until combined.
- Add in 1 tablespoon of water at a time until the mixture is wet enough to roll out as dough.

- Roll out dough and cut shapes with your pet-themed or other favorite cookie cutters.
- Place onto cookie sheet.
- Bake for 20 minutes.
- Let cool and place in a decorated shoebox or other container (use pictures of pets from magazines to decorate).

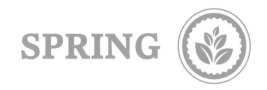

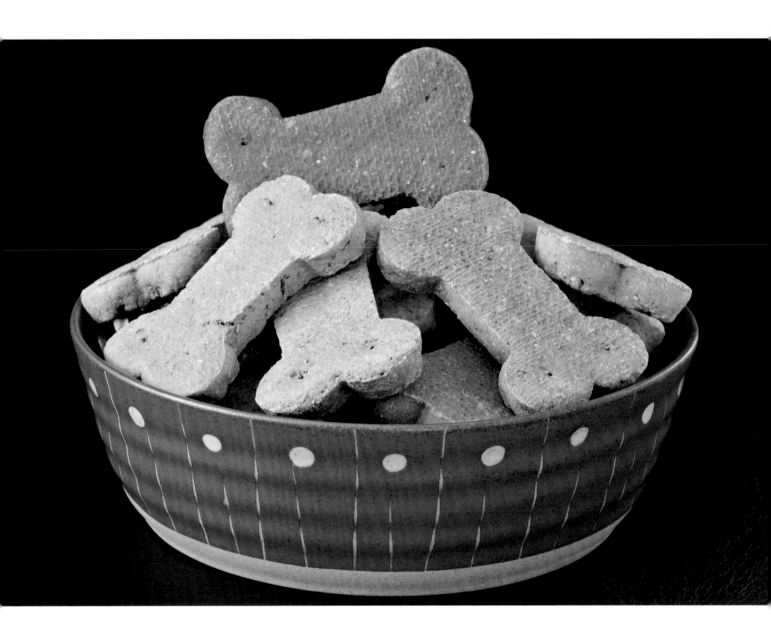

▸ Did you ever grow a garden? What kind of garden (vegetable, herb, flower)?

▸ How big was your garden? Was it a large garden or a smaller one, such as a window garden or planter?

▸ What are your favorite things about gardens?

▸ Did you ever visit a famous garden? What do you remember about it?

▸ What kinds of insects are found in a garden? (Worms, ladybugs, praying mantises, snails, spiders, potato bugs, aphids, slugs, etc.)

▸ Let's name some things that we eat that grow in a garden. (For instance, tomatoes, squash, peas, beans, berries, lettuce, cucumbers, potatoes, onions, herbs, and eggplants.)

▸ Have you ever visited a farm? What do you remember about it?

▸ What are some crops that grow on a farm? (Corn, wheat, rye, potatoes, etc.)

▸ What kinds of tools are used in a garden? (Hoe, rake, watering hose, stakes, shovel, spade, bulb planter, pruning shears, trowel, etc.)

LET'S TRY . . .

▸ Putting together a gardening toolkit with objects commonly used in gardening, such as gardening tools, gardening gloves, seed packets, and a watering can. Talk about each of the objects, how they are used and what they are used for.

▸ Watching gardening shows together on TV.

▸ Planting grass seed in a small container to grow in your setting.

▸ Looking at books or magazines with photographs of gardens together, including famous gardens of the world, such as Versailles (France), Boboli Gardens (Italy), Tivoli Gardens (Netherlands), Butchart Gardens (Canada), and the White House Rose Garden (United States).

▸ Planting an herb container garden using fragrant herbs. (Rosemary, chives, etc.)

▸ Visiting a local community garden, garden center, or farm together. Talk about all the tools, buildings, plantings, and colors of the plants that you see.

▸ Playing a seed-packet matching game. Buy 12 seed packets, 2 of each kind (for example, 2 tomato, 2 cucumber, and 2 squash). You will have 6 different pairs of seed packets. Next, put 6 packets on a table. Work together to match the remaining 6 seed packets with the ones on the table, matching one at a time. Talk about each packet (the color, how the seeds are planted, what you can do with the vegetables that grow from them, etc.). Try to pick packets of their favorite vegetables or herbs.

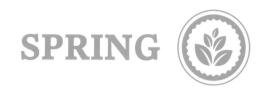

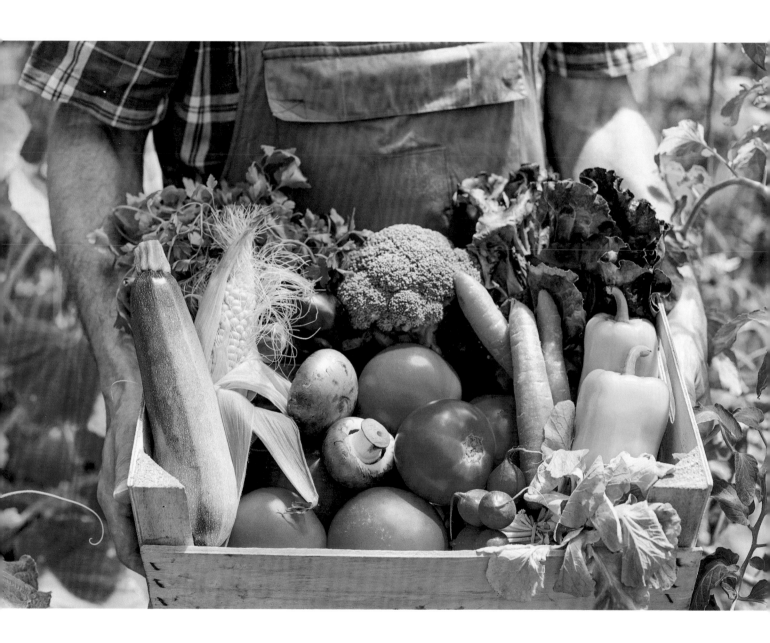

Gardens come to life in the spring.

LET'S MAKE A SWEET POTATO VINE

Growing a sweet potato vine is an easy and enjoyable activity you can share.

You Will Need:

- 1 small sweet potato
- Several toothpicks
- Small plastic cup or jar
- Water, enough to fill the cup or jar three-quarters of the way full

Instructions

- Fill the plastic cup or jar with water.
- Place the toothpicks together around the middle of the sweet potato, one on each side. Place the sweet potato in the plastic cup so that it is suspended by the toothpicks on the rim of the cup with half of the potato resting in the water.
- Place the sweet potato in a sunny location. Over several days roots will sprout.
- You can then plant the sweet potato in a container or outside in the garden and grow a sweet potato vine.

See also https://extension.illinois.edu/gpe/case5/c5hgi.html.

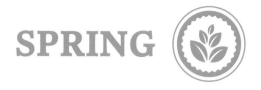

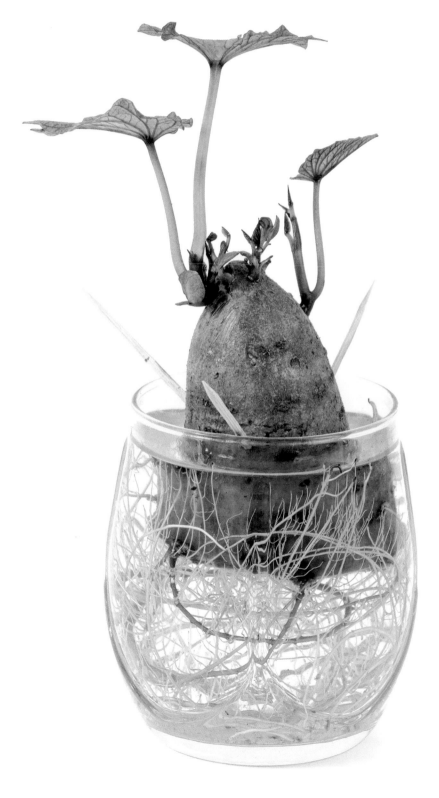

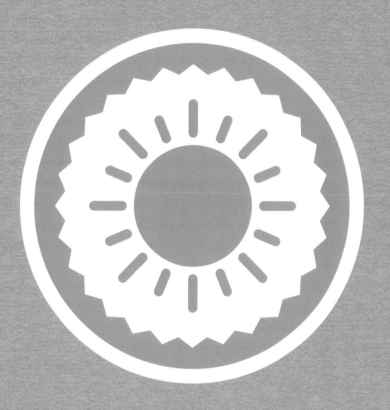

SUMMER

LET'S TALK ABOUT ...

- What did you like to play outside when you were young?

- Did you have a favorite place to play outside when you were a child?

- What sounds do children make when they play?

- How do you feel when you hear children laughing?

- What other sounds do we hear outside in summer?

- Did you ever go to camp? Where did you go to camp? Did you like camp?

LET'S TRY ...

- Watching children play on a playground or at a park.

- Talking about memories of playing games like hopscotch or jacks.

- Playing some outside games, such as rolling a ball to each other or having a gentle game of catch.

- Having a beanbag toss or playing games like tic-tac-toe.

- If possible, providing interaction with young children to play some gentle games.

- Swinging gently on a porch swing.

- Teaching a simple game to a grandchild or child if you are able to.

- Making a games memory box. Put familiar outdoor game objects, such as balls, jacks, sidewalk chalk, marbles, and so on, in a shoebox. You can use the objects in the box to look at and talk about childhood memories. If you'd like, you can decorate the shoebox using wrapping paper or magazine photos with game-themed images.

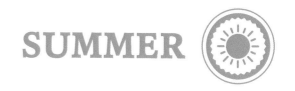

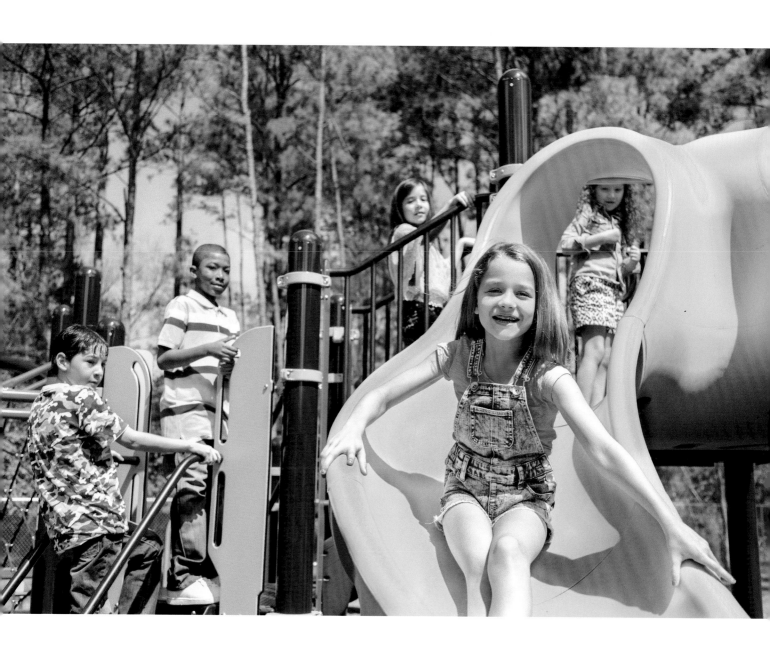

I like to watch the children play outside.

LET'S TALK ABOUT . . .

- What is your favorite flavor of ice cream?

- Do you like to eat your ice cream from a cone or a cup? Why?

- What are your favorite ice-cream toppings?

- Did you ever make ice cream? How did you do it?

- Where would you eat ice cream in the summer? At the beach? On the front porch? At a favorite ice-cream stand?

- What are your favorite ice-cream treats? Ice-cream sandwiches, sundaes, banana splits, ice-cream sodas?

LET'S TRY . . .

- Tasting different flavors of ice cream together.

- Making homemade ice cream, an ice-cream cake, or freezer popsicles.

- Making sundaes, banana splits, or ice-cream sodas.

- Visiting an ice-cream parlor together.

- Having an ice-cream-parlor party with family and friends. Make old-fashioned ice-cream treats, such as malted milk-shakes, ice-cream sodas, and egg creams.

- Naming different flavors of ice cream together.

- Reading some poems about ice cream together. You can find poems on websites such as www.poets.org or www.poetry foundation.org.

- Singing songs about ice cream or summer together, such as "Lazy Days of Summer," "Save Your Heart for Me," "In the Summer-time," and other similar songs.

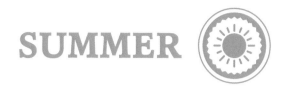

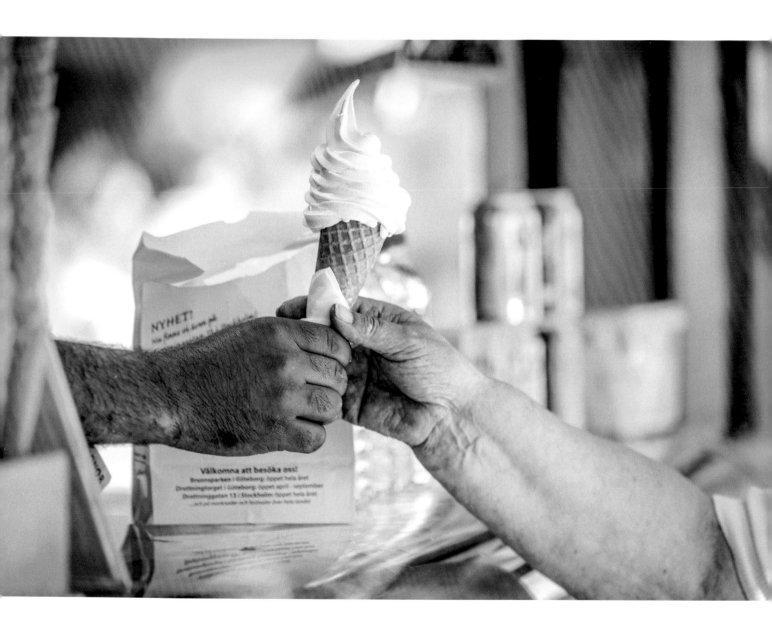

Ice cream tastes good on a hot summer day.

LET'S MAKE ICE CREAM IN A BAG

This fun and simple activity results in a delicious treat to share together. Make one bag per person. Try topping with fresh fruit or chopped nuts.

You Will Need (per bag of ice cream):

- 1 tablespoon sugar
- ½ cup whole milk
- ¼ teaspoon vanilla extract
- 5 cups ice (*approximately*)
- 6 tablespoons kosher salt

- 1 quart-sized resealable zippered plastic bag
- 1 gallon-sized resealable zippered plastic bag
- 1 kitchen cloth

Instructions

- Place the whole milk, vanilla extract, and sugar into the quart-sized plastic bag and seal the bag.
- Next, fill the gallon-sized bag half full with ice and add the salt.
- Place the quart-sized bag inside the gallon-sized bag and seal the bag.

- Shake until mixture is the consistency of ice cream, about 5 minutes. If the bag becomes too cold to handle, use the kitchen cloth for insulation.
- Remove the quart-sized bag from the gallon-sized bag.
- Empty the ice cream into a dish. Add desired toppings and enjoy!

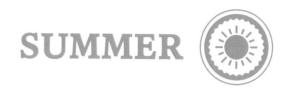

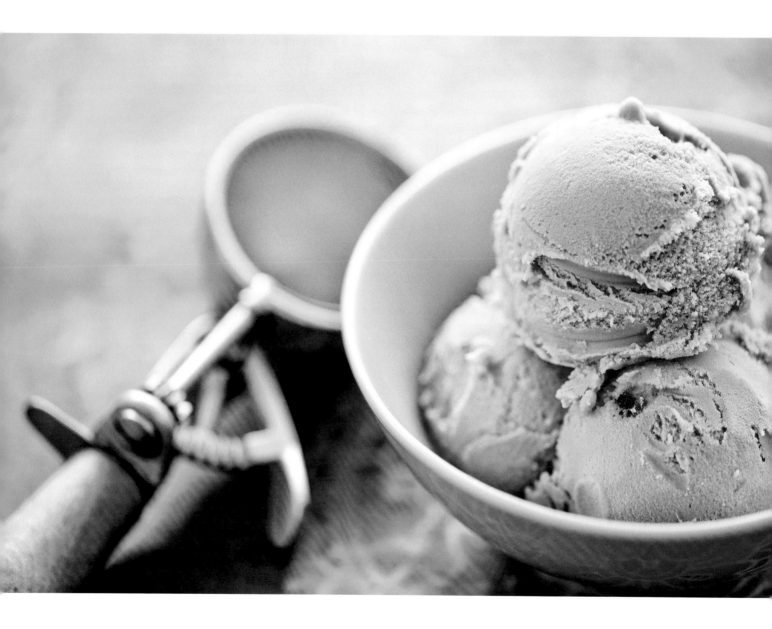

LET'S TALK ABOUT . . .

- Do you like picnics?

- What kinds of foods do you bring on picnics?

- What are your favorite picnic foods?

- Did your family have a special picnic tradition? Did you picnic on holidays or have special picnic foods you made?

- Do you remember any special picnics, such as a family reunion or celebration?

- Do you like to eat barbecue? What kinds of foods do you like cooked on a barbecue?

- Did you ever cook food over a campfire? What did you cook?

LET'S TRY . . .

- Having a picnic with family or friends. Use a picnic cloth and picnic basket. Prepare typical picnic foods, such as cucumber salad, potato salad, egg salad, cheeses, sandwiches, fruit salad, chips, watermelon, and cookies.

- Tasting different condiments used at a barbecue, such as ketchup, mustard, relish, and barbecue sauce.

- Tasting typical picnic or barbecue foods from other cultures, such as France, Mexico, or India.

- Looking at cookbooks for picnic recipes together.

- Making a potato or egg salad. Have everything washed and cut up ahead of time so that you can mix the ingredients together.

- Making a collage using photographs of favorite picnic foods and picnic scenes.

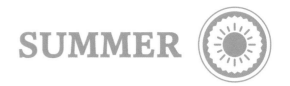

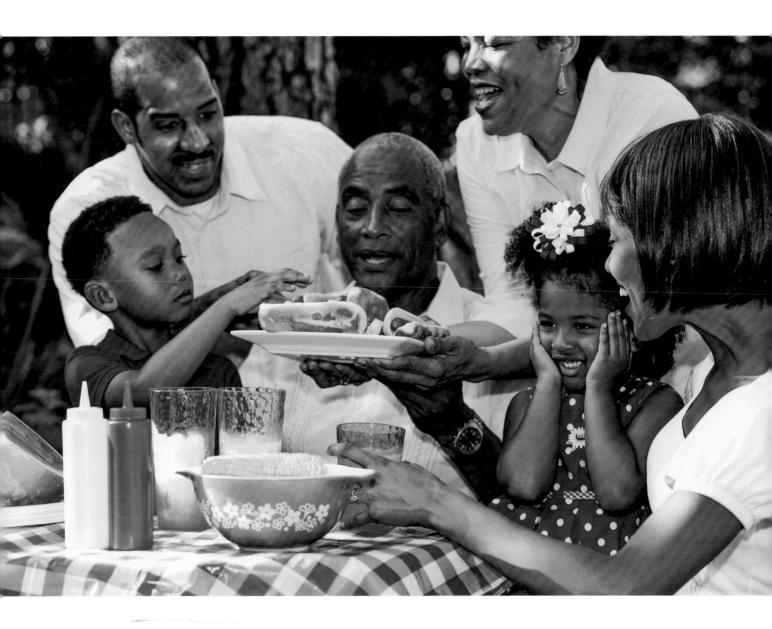

I like sharing picnics with family and friends.

LET'S TALK ABOUT ...

- What kinds of fruits do you like?

- Let's see how many different fruits we can name.

- What are your favorite foods made with fruit? (Offer prompts by naming fruit-based foods, such as applesauce, banana bread, cherry pie, plum tart, etc.)

- Did you ever visit an orchard or pick berries? Can you tell me about it?

- Do you have a favorite recipe containing fruit? What is in it?

- Do you like fruit juices? Which is your favorite?

- Let's see how many red fruits we can think of together. How many yellow fruits? (You can repeat this with other colors, such as orange, green, etc.)

LET'S TRY ...

- Making a fruit salad together using seasonal fresh fruit.

- Singing songs that reference different fruits, such as "Don't Sit Under the Apple Tree," "Yes! We Have No Bananas," "Billy Boy," and "Lemon Tree."

- Making art prints using fruit and non-toxic paint. Use sturdy fruits, such as peaches, apples, and lemons. Cut the fruit in half lengthwise. Help the person dip the cut side of the fruit into the paint and then press the fruit gently on the paper. Repeat these steps as desired to create a custom fruit print.

- Having a "fruit-water" tasting. Take different fresh fruits, such as lemons, limes, oranges, apples, berries, and the like, and add them to cool still or sparkling water. You can create single-fruit flavors or combine different fruits. Taste the waters together, talking about how they taste and which ones you like best.

- Making "rock" fruit. You will need small, clean, and smooth rocks in round or oblong shapes, nontoxic paints of varying colors, and paint brushes of different sizes. Work together to paint the rocks to resemble different fruits.

- Visiting a farm and picking berries together.

- Going to a farmer's market or grocery store, shopping for and talking about the different fruits and fruit products.

- Tasting the same fruit prepared in different ways and comparing how they taste. Discuss which you like better. For example, you can try fresh grapes, raisins, grape juice, and grape fruit leather.

- Playing with fruit pits. Save and clean pits from different fruits. Study the pits together and see if you can identify which fruit they are from. Talk about the different size, color, and shape of the pits and how they feel.

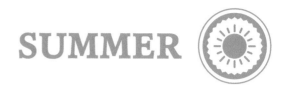

SUMMER

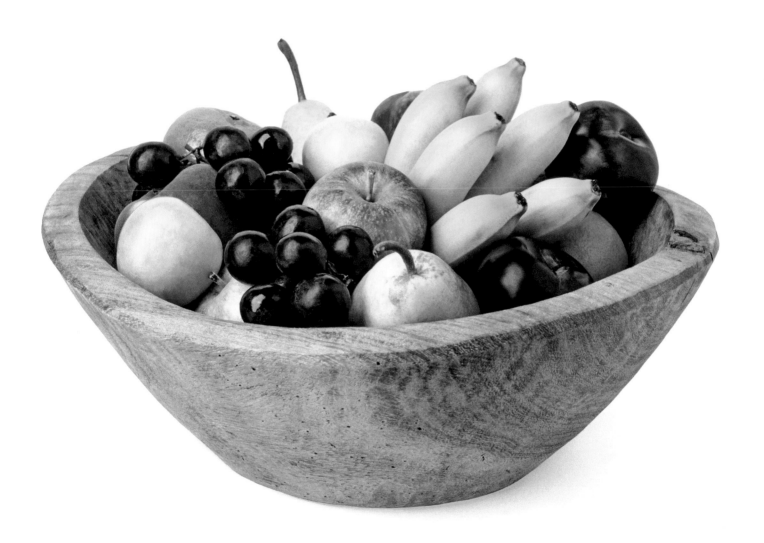

Summer fruits are sweet and juicy.

LET'S MAKE A FRUIT SMOOTHIE

Smoothies are a popular way to have a nutritious snack or morning meal. Use different fruits for an endless variety of smoothie recipes.

You Will Need:

- 1 quart berries, washed, pitted, and cleaned as needed
- 1 ripe banana, broken into chunks
- 2 peaches or other stone fruit, peeled, pitted, and cut into chunks

- 2 cups ice
- Blender
- Glasses
- Straws

Other Smoothie Ingredients You Can Add:

- Vanilla or plain yogurt
- Orange juice
- Fresh dark greens, such as spinach or kale (freezing the greens and then adding them will help them blend into the smoothie)

- Cocoa powder
- Nut butter, such as peanut or almond butter

Instructions

- Place all the items except the ice into a blender and puree for about 1 minute.
- Add the ice in two batches, blending each time you add more ice.

- Blend to desired consistency.
- Pour into glasses and serve with straws.

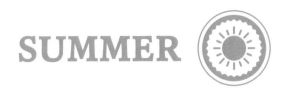

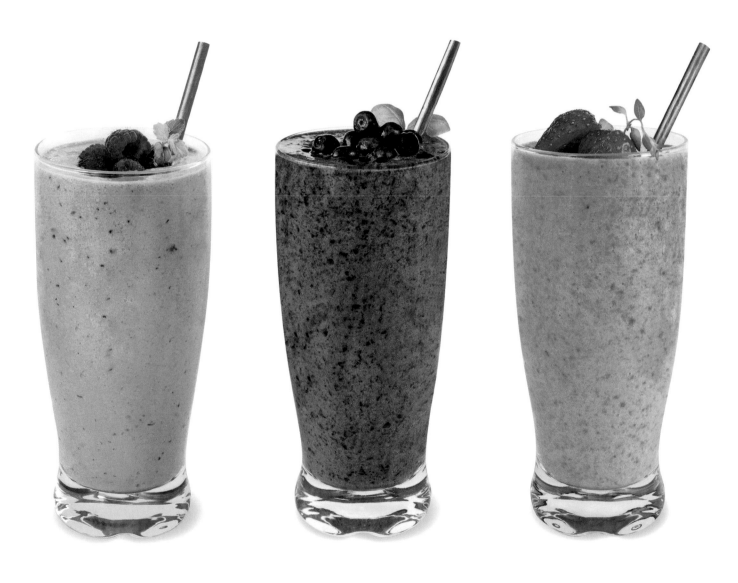

▸ Do you like baseball? What other sports do you like?

▸ What are the different things you need to play baseball? (Talk about the different equipment needed to play the game, such as bats, balls, bases, etc.)

▸ Do you remember some famous baseball players? What do you remember about them?

▸ What other sports are played in the summer?

▸ Did you ever go to a baseball game? What can you tell me about it?

▸ Going to a baseball game together.

▸ Visiting a local baseball field. Walk around the bases, sit in the bleachers, and so on.

▸ Watching videos of old baseball-game highlights or full games. You can find them online or rent them from your local library.

▸ Playing a gentle game of catch with a foam ball.

▸ Decorating baseball caps using fabric markers, patches from favorite baseball teams, and press-on letters. (You can find these materials at your local crafts store.)

▸ Having a baseball-themed party. Use paper goods decorated with baseball themes. Serve foods typically found at a ballpark, such as hot dogs, soft pretzels, sodas, and ice cream. Play baseball songs or have baseball movies playing in the background.

▸ Reading "Casey at the Bat" together (*see page 94*). Talk about what is happening in the poem as you read it, acting out different parts of the poem if you are able to.

▸ Watching classic films about baseball, such as *Damn Yankees*, *Field of Dreams*, *Bull Durham*, or *A League of Their Own*.

▸ Looking at old baseball cards together. You can find books with images of old baseball cards, look at them online, or visit a store that sells baseball cards or sports memorabilia.

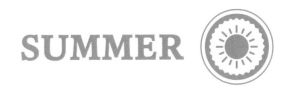

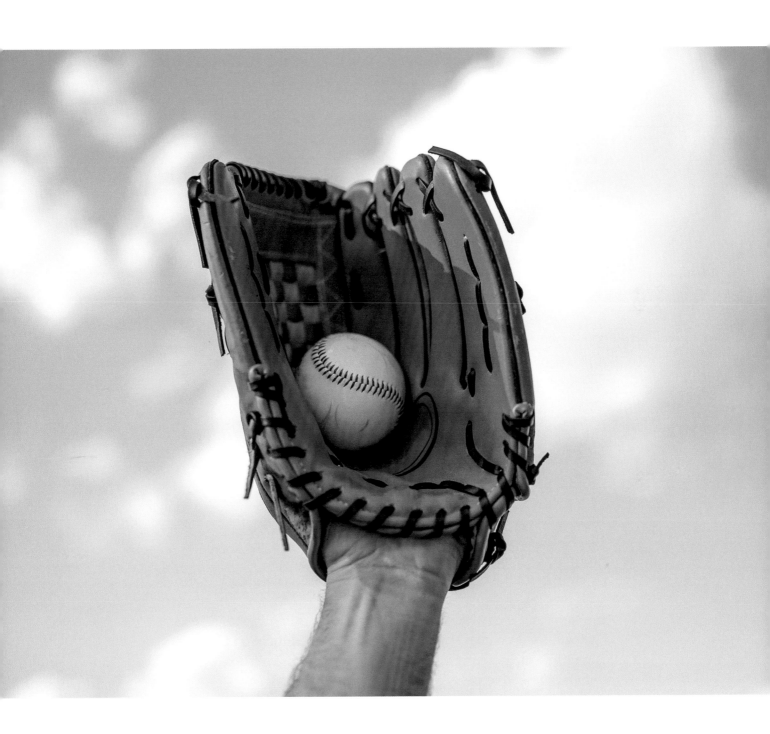

Baseball is fun to watch and play.

Casey at the Bat
Ernest Lawrence Thayer

The outlook wasn't brilliant for the Mudville nine that day:
The score stood four to two, with but one inning more to play,
And then when Cooney died at first, and Barrows did the same,
A pall-like silence fell upon the patrons of the game.

A straggling few got up to go in deep despair. The rest
Clung to the hope which springs eternal in the human breast;
They thought, "If only Casey could but get a whack at that—
We'd put up even money now, with Casey at the bat."

But Flynn preceded Casey, as did also Jimmy Blake,
And the former was a hoodoo, while the latter was a cake;
So upon that stricken multitude grim melancholy sat,
For there seemed but little chance of Casey getting to the bat.

But Flynn let drive a single, to the wonderment of all,
And Blake, the much despisèd, tore the cover off the ball;
And when the dust had lifted, and men saw what had occurred,
There was Jimmy safe at second and Flynn a-hugging third.

Then from five thousand throats and more there rose a lusty yell;
It rumbled through the valley, it rattled in the dell;
It pounded on the mountain and recoiled upon the flat,
For Casey, mighty Casey, was advancing to the bat.

There was ease in Casey's manner as he stepped into his place;
There was pride in Casey's bearing and a smile lit Casey's face.
And when, responding to the cheers, he lightly doffed his hat,
No stranger in the crowd could doubt 'twas Casey at the bat.

Ten thousand eyes were on him as he rubbed his hands with dirt;
Five thousand tongues applauded when he wiped them on his shirt;
Then while the writhing pitcher ground the ball into his hip,
Defiance flashed in Casey's eye, a sneer curled Casey's lip.

And now the leather-covered sphere came hurtling through the air,
And Casey stood a-watching it in haughty grandeur there.
Close by the sturdy batsman the ball unheeded sped—
"That ain't my style," said Casey. "Strike one!" the umpire said.

From the benches, black with people, there went up a muffled roar,
Like the beating of the storm-waves on a stern and distant shore;
"Kill him! Kill the umpire!" shouted someone on the stand;
And it's likely they'd have killed him had not Casey raised his hand.

With a smile of Christian charity great Casey's visage shone;
He stilled the rising tumult; he bade the game go on;
He signaled to the pitcher, and once more the dun sphere flew;
But Casey still ignored it and the umpire said, "Strike two!"

"Fraud!" cried the maddened thousands, and echo answered "Fraud!"
But one scornful look from Casey and the audience was awed.
They saw his face grow stern and cold, they saw his muscles strain,
And they knew that Casey wouldn't let that ball go by again.

The sneer is gone from Casey's lip, his teeth are clenched in hate,
He pounds with cruel violence his bat upon the plate;
And now the pitcher holds the ball, and now he lets it go,
And now the air is shattered by the force of Casey's blow.

Oh, somewhere in this favoured land the sun is shining bright,
The band is playing somewhere, and somewhere hearts are light;
And somewhere men are laughing, and somewhere children shout,
But there is no joy in Mudville—mighty Casey has struck out.

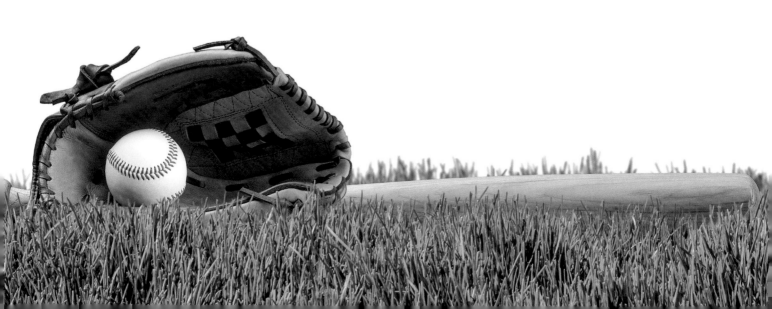

LET'S TALK ABOUT . . .

- Do you know how to swim?

- How old were you when you learned to swim? Who taught you how to swim?

- Did you like to swim in a pool, lake, or ocean?

- Do you like to float on your back?

- What types of swimming strokes can you do? Can you do the backstroke, crawl, or breaststroke?

- Were you ever on a swim team? Did you ever participate in a swim race?

- What kinds of games did you play in the water?

- What did your favorite bathing suit look like?

- Did you ever see the fish swimming around your feet in a lake or ocean?

LET'S TRY . . .

- Going to a local pool for a swim.

- Watching a swim race at the local high school or on TV.

- "Practicing" our swimming strokes by moving our arms and legs to mimic different strokes. (You can do this while seated.)

- Talking about famous swimmers, such as Esther Williams, Johnny Weissmuller, Mark Spitz, Michael Phelps, and Diana Nyad.

- Taking a beginner's pool-exercise class together.

- Watching a swimming-themed movie, such as *Dangerous When Wet* or *Million Dollar Mermaid*.

- Reading about Esther Williams and looking at photographs of her on the internet together.

- Visiting local lakes to have a picnic and watch the swimmers.

- Making a collage of different swimsuits from photos cut out of magazines or printed from the internet.

- Purchasing fish and a small fish tank. Set up the tank together and then spend time watching and caring for the fish together.

- Visiting a local aquarium to see the different fish and aquatic species there.

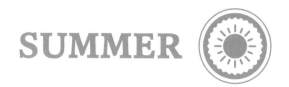

SUMMER

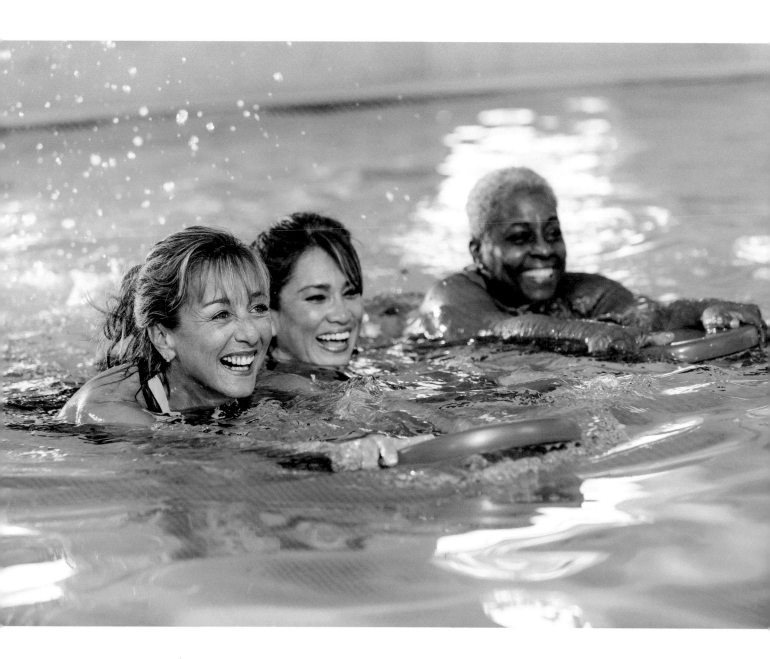

Swimming is fun when it is hot outside.

LET'S TALK ABOUT . . .

- What is your favorite thing to do at a fair?

- Did you ever enter a contest at a county fair, like a pie-eating contest?

- Did you ever raise an animal to enter in a fair, such as a pig, chicken, or calf?

- What were your favorite rides at the fair?

- What were your favorite games to play at the fair? Did you ever win anything?

- Did you ever go to a street fair or carnival? Can you tell me about it?

- Did you ever go to an unusual fair, like a book or art fair? A world's fair? What do you remember about it?

- Who would you go to a fair with?

- What foods would you eat at a fair?

LET'S TRY . . .

- Naming and talking about the different kinds of fairs or carnivals, such as county, street, art, book, and holiday fairs.

- Making a pudding pie. You can purchase a ready-made pie shell and fill it with chocolate, vanilla, or banana pudding.

- Playing "Ring the Wind Chimes." Hang wind chimes from the ceiling and toss a beach ball to make them ring.

- Holding your own carnival for family and friends. Play games you might find at a fair, such as ring toss, bowling, or cornhole (you can find additional carnival game ideas online). Serve typical fair foods, such as soft pretzels, cotton candy, caramel popcorn, pizza, ice-cream sandwiches, and others.

- Having a photo booth. Gather fun hats, scarves, glasses, and other costume items. Dress up with the different costume items and take photos together using a smartphone or camera.

- Visiting a local fair or carnival together. Look for a street, county, arts and crafts, or book fair to attend.

- Watching a classic movie together that features carnivals or fairs, such as *Dumbo*, *The Greatest Show on Earth*, *Carousel*, or *Roustabout*.

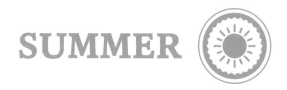

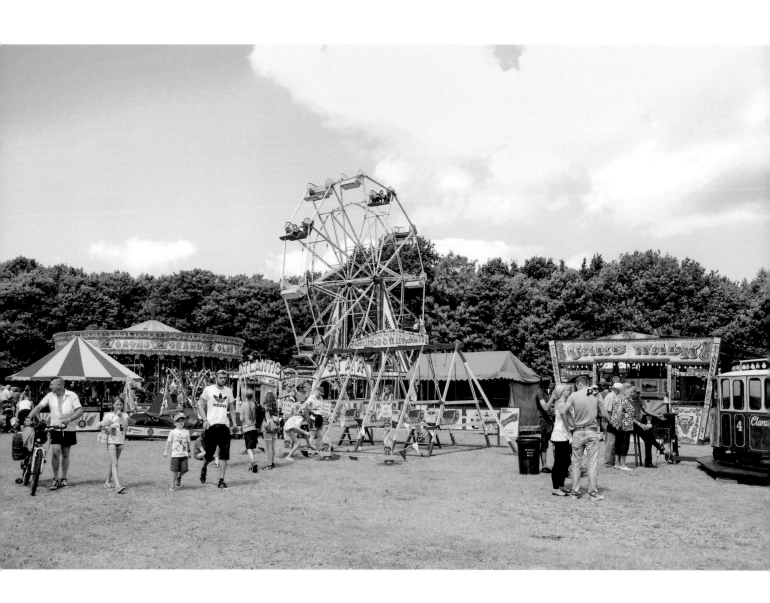

There is always a lot to do at a fair.

LET'S TALK ABOUT . . .

- Have you visited the beach in summer? Where did you go to the beach?

- What are the sounds we hear at the beach?

- What kinds of things do we find in the sand?

- How does the sand feel on your feet at the beach?

- Do you like to go for walks on the beach?

- Do you like to swim in the ocean?

- What kinds of games would you play at the beach?

- What would you take to the beach? Do you like to sit on a chair or towel at the beach? Would you use an umbrella?

- How do the sounds of the ocean make you feel?

LET'S TRY . . .

- Making a sand-art project. (You can find sand-art kits at most crafts stores.)

- Buying a bag of sand and warming it in the sun. Then try touching the sand together, running it through your fingers and putting your bare feet in it. Talk about how it feels.

- Making a keepsake beach box. Use a shoe-box or other cardboard box. Decorate it with paint or pictures of the seashore cut from magazines. Inside the box put sand, seashells, and other objects you can find at the beach.

- Listening to a recording of ocean sounds.

- Watching old movies with a beach theme, such as *Beach Party*, *Beach Blanket Bingo*, *Gidget*, and so on.

- Taking a walk at the beach, either on the sand or on a boardwalk.

- Getting a conch shell and listening to the sounds when we put it to our ears.

- Visiting a lighthouse.

- Looking at photos of beaches or beach scenes together. You can find photos online or books of beach photos at your local library.

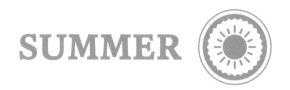

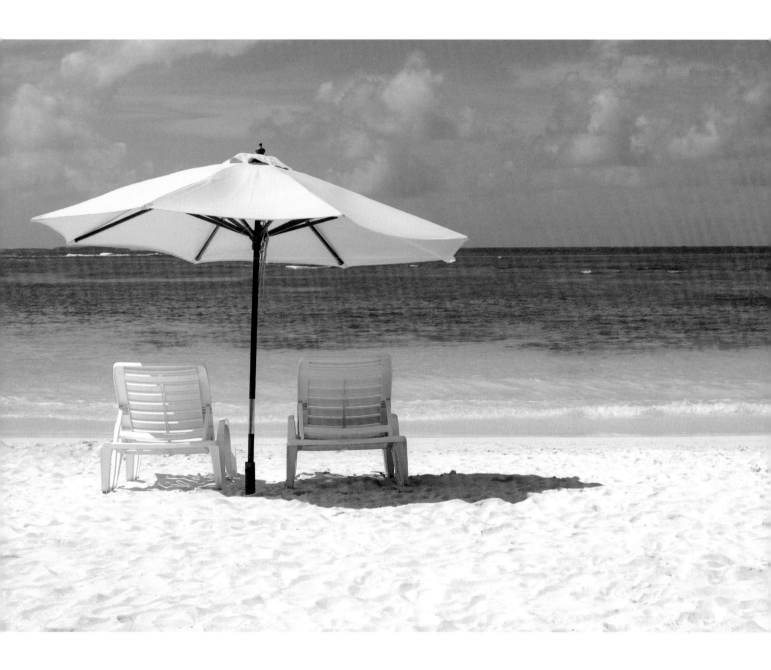

The sounds at the beach make me happy.

RESOURCES FOR CAREGIVERS

ORGANIZATIONS AND ASSOCIATIONS

Numerous organizations and associations offer information for individuals living with dementia and their care partners.

Alzheimer's Association
(800) 272-3900
www.alz.org

With 300 chapters across the United States offering caregiver support, education, and resources, the Alzheimer's Association is the largest US nonprofit association supporting individuals and families affected by Alzheimer disease and related memory disorders.

Alzheimer's Foundation of America
(866) 232-8484
www.alzfdn.org

The Alzheimer's Foundation of America provides information about how to care for people with Alzheimer's, as well as a list of services for people with the disease, including a toll-free hotline, publications, and other educational materials.

Eldercare Locator
(800) 677-1116
www.eldercare.gov

A service of the Administration on Aging, Eldercare Locator is a clearinghouse for information on community resources, including home care, adult day care, and nursing homes.

Family Caregiver Alliance
(800) 445-8106
www.caregiver.org

The Family Caregiver Alliance is a community-based nonprofit organization offering support services for those caring for adults with neurological disorders including Alzheimer disease, stroke, and traumatic brain injury.

National Institute on Aging (NIH) Alzheimer's Caregiving Website
(800) 222-2225
https://www.nia.nih.gov/health/alzheimers/caregiving

The National Institute on Aging's Alzheimer's Caregiving Information provides caregivers with information on and useful tools for daily care.

Alzheimer's and Related Dementias Education and Referral (ADEAR) Center
(800) 438-4380
https://www.nia.nih.gov/alzheimers

The ADEAR Center offers information on diagnosis, treatment, patient care, caregiver needs, long-term care, and research and clinical trials related to Alzheimer disease.

The Simon Foundation for Continence
(800) 237-4666
www.simonfoundation.org

Support and resources for individuals with incontinence, as well as their families and health professionals.

Dementia Action Alliance USA
(732) 212-9036
http://daanow.org

The Dementia Action Alliance USA is a non-profit advocacy and education organization for people living with dementia, their care partners, friends, and dementia specialists looking to improve the experience of living with dementia in the United States.

PUBLICATIONS AND ARTICLES

Numerous publications are available that can be helpful in understanding more about memory disorders and the caregiving experience.

The 36-Hour Day: A Family Guide for People Who Have Alzheimer Disease, Other Dementias, and Memory Loss, 6th Edition
Nancy L. Mace, MA, and Peter V. Rabins, MD, MPH
Baltimore: Johns Hopkins University Press, 2017.

This classic text offers information on all aspects of caring for a loved one with dementia. It covers information on the disease process, living arrangements, financial and legal considerations, daily care, medications, mood, and other behavioral changes.

"Living with Dementia:
Changing the Status Quo"
Dementia Action Alliance, 2016.
https://daanow.org/wp-content/uploads
/2016/04/Living_Fully_With_Dementia
_White-Paper_040316.pdf

This white paper from a leading dementia advocacy group outlines how we can reframe how we see dementia to improve the experience of living with memory loss for the individual, their care partners, and communities.

"Words Matter: See Me, Not My Dementia"
Dementia Action Alliance, 2015.
https://daanow.org/wp-content/uploads
/2016/03/Words_Matter-See-Me-Not-My
-Dementia.pdf

A powerful reminder of how words matter in our interactions, with helpful guidelines to using more positive language in the service of reducing stigma and misperceptions regarding dementia and those affected by memory challenge.

ABOUT THE AUTHORS

CYNTHIA R. GREEN, PhD, is a clinical psychologist who is a leading expert and author in the field of brain health. Dr. Green is the CEO of TBH Brands, the parent company of Total Brain Health, a leading provider of training products and services to improve memory and brain fitness. Core products of Total Brain Health include the Total Brain Health® Toolkits line, a series of "programs in a box" designed for use in active aging, fitness, and wellness settings. A member of the Department of Psychiatry faculty at the Mount Sinai School of Medicine since 1990, Dr. Green is the author of 5 books on brain health, both on her own and in collaboration with major brands such as Prevention and National Geographic. Her book with National Geographic, *Your Best Brain Ever*, was named a "2013 Top Guide to Life After 50" by the *Wall Street Journal*. In addition, Dr. Green frequently serves as a consultant to companies on memory and brain fitness and is a highly regarded keynote speaker for organizational, corporate, and association events. Dr. Green is a regular media guest whose work has been featured on *Dr. Oz, Good Morning America, 20/20, CNBC, Fox,* and *The Martha Stewart Show*, as well as in *Time, Newsweek, The New York Times, The Washington Post,* and *Good Housekeeping*. Originally from North Carolina, Dr. Green lives with her family in northern New Jersey.

JOAN BELOFF, ACC, ALA, CDP, is a specialist in the field of gerontology, with more than thirty years of experience. Ms. Beloff currently serves as the Chief Development Officer for Chilton Medical Center in Pompton Plains, New Jersey, and provides oversight for the New Vitality and Community Outreach programs. New Vitality is a health and wellness program for adults 65 and older. She served as nominations chairperson for the National Association of Activity Professionals, Eastern Region, and is a past president of the Society on Aging of New Jersey. Ms. Beloff has been honored for her innovative educational programs by the Catalyst Institute for Innovation and Excellence and by the Wayne Alliance for the Prevention of Drug and Alcohol Abuse. Ms. Beloff also received an award from the National Council on Aging for "Best Health Promotion Practice" for the New Vitality program. Ms. Beloff is licensed in the state of New Jersey as an Assisted Living Administrator and has spoken both locally and nationally on aging issues.

Both Dr. Green and Ms. Beloff regularly present at national conferences on aging and senior health. They have collaborated for many years on programs addressing memory wellness and senior health issues. They received the New Jersey Partners for Success award from the New Jersey Partners in Aging, Mental Health and Substance Abuse for their innovative program on memory and alcohol abuse, "Keep Your Memory Sharp! Tips for Success."